Exhale Weight
Breathe a sigh of relief, it's time to let go
By Jo-Anne Eadie

ISBN-13: 978-1539118763
ISBN-10: 1539118762

4th Edition Printed in Canada | 2016

Author's Disclaimer:

I am not a Doctor, Nutritionist, or educated in any Medical, Scientific, or Biological Training. I am not a Personal Trainer or Coach. I have training and degrees in Hypnosis, EFT, NLP and weight solutions.

This book contains personal experiences only, with my own weight journey, and my clients who have come to me for Hypnosis and/or EFT to help gain control of their weight.

I think I have purchased, read and tried just about every diet book on the market and have sorted out a lot of what works and what doesn't for myself and many of my clients.

Since I am not an "expert", I did not include all information on all the topics that I could have. There are many topics touched upon in this book that you can easily look up online yourself if you want a more thorough explanation.

All the things in this book have been gathered over the years from my own journey. I can't even remember where some of it came from.

I kept what worked and let go of what didn't.

Exhale Weight

Breathe a sigh of relief, It's time to let go

Jo-Anne Eadie

Board Certified, Master Consulting Hypnotist
Virtual Gastric Band with Hypnosis Practitioner
Licenced, Certified Trainer - Virtual Gastric Band with Hypnosis
Pioneered by Sheila Granger

NGH Certified Hypnosis Instructor
EFT-Certified-1

Common Sense

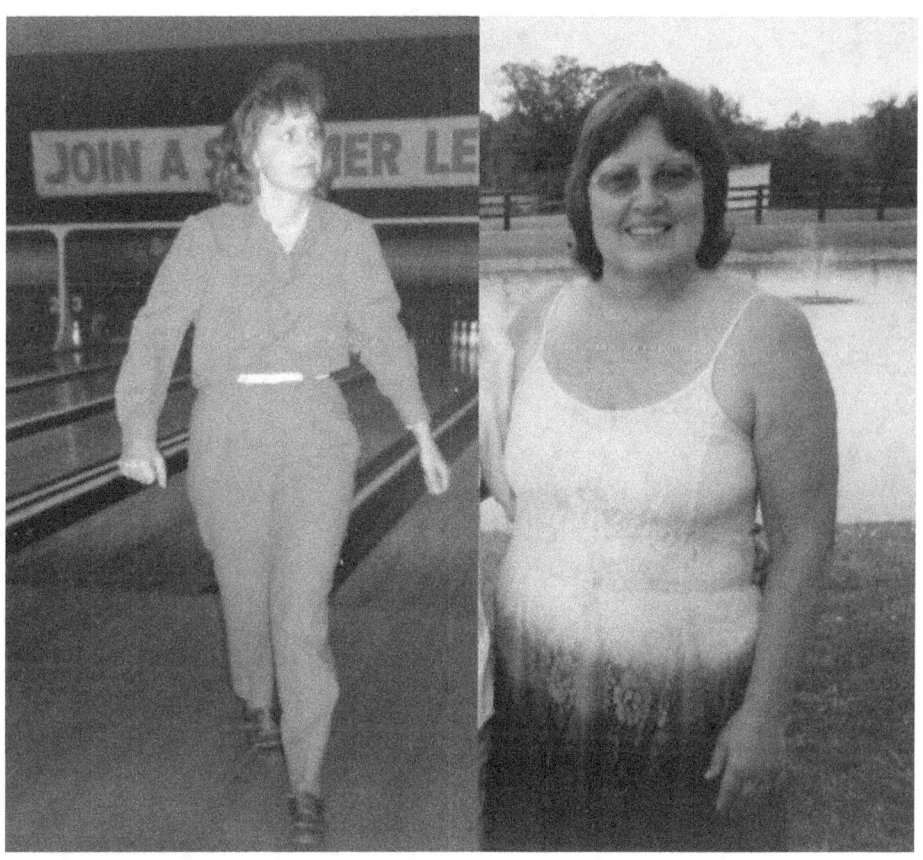

So thin that my husband bought a
product called Wate On

In middle age, 50 pounds
visited and would not leave

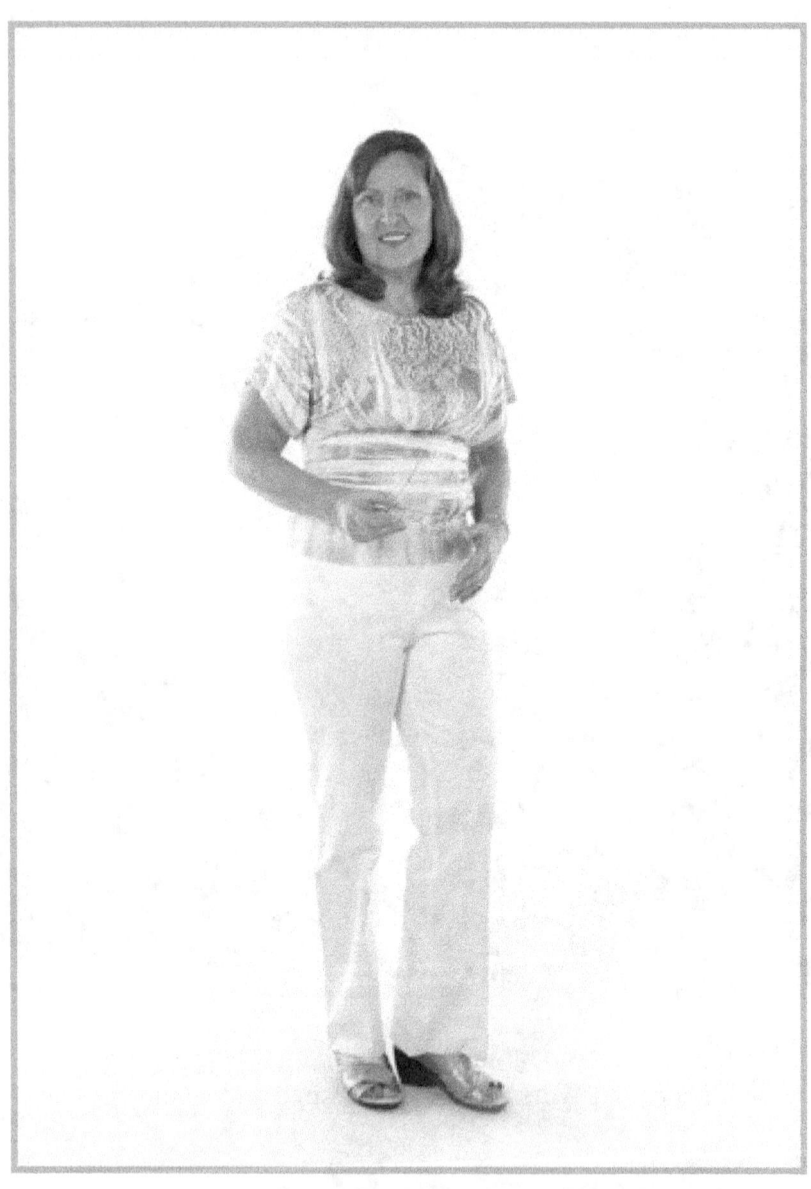

I am a practitioner of the Virtual Gastric Band, and also a client. This is the way I will be for the rest of my life. Not a diet, but a lifestyle change.

Power of Freedom

My company is called "Power of Freedom"- When you find emotional freedom, you gain your own personal power.

It is a journey that has taken me a long time and a lot of work; and the rewards are wonderful. I think it is a journey that never ends.

I now just live for today and tackle what comes up in the now.

I love helping my clients move forward on their journey and value the uniqueness each client brings to their sessions. It is the most interesting and fulfilling work imaginable.

Significance of the Infinity Sign

The infinity sign means forever and I am always hopeful that for my clients, the work I do with them to move forward is forever.

If they always walk out of my door feeling better than when they walked in, I am fulfilled

Table of Contents

Page #

*I am in total control of
what I eat,
when I eat
and how much I eat!*

I am in total control

Part One:
Introduction

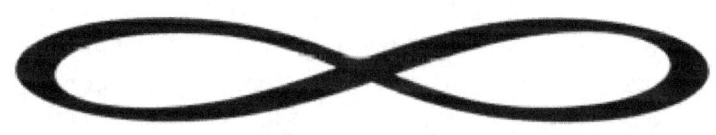

I'm so grateful I'm creating really favourable things to happen for myself today and for others.

Recollections from the Past

As a child, I was tall and thin and could eat anything I wanted, as much as I wanted, whenever I wanted and never gain a pound. I obviously ate large amounts of food as relatives, friends and acquaintances around me commented about me having a hollow leg and growing like a weed. **Such affirming comments!** When I hit middle age and menopause, fifty extra pounds gradually visited and stayed and I began this journey of trying to get them to leave.

If you have had considered yourself overweight all your life, you may be lacking sympathy for someone who writes that most of her life she could eat whatever she wanted. Trying to compare someone who has watched what they ate for years and someone who just began to do that in middle age is apples and oranges. Both are unique to find a solution that works.

I have a lifelong sugar addiction. I didn't realize this until the weight began to stay on me once I turned fifty. In trying to release weight, I have become aware that perceived stress would send me to eating something sweet. **Once I knew, I couldn't pretend I didn't know.**

I have found various important times when the behaviours I sometimes find myself doing today have definite roots from my childhood.

My Mother was always home when I came home from school until I was 12 or 13 when she got a part time job and we came home to an empty house. My brothers went out to feed the calves and do the chores in the barn. My older sister didn't get home from High School until later.

I don't remember this happening when my Mother was home. When the house was empty, I was ravenously hungry and I would eat and eat and eat after school. My Mother had left dinner half prepared and I was to finish it and have it on the table precisely at six o'clock when

10

my father, sister and brothers all came in. Sometimes on those days I had eaten so much, I picked at my dinner and had to force myself to eat or "they" would find out I had gorged myself on too many snacks.

At one of the courses I was taking, a lady stood up and protested that she had come from a dysfunctional childhood. The Instructor asked for a show of hands of how many people in the class had a happy, fulfilled childhood with loving parents. One person put up their hand. Once you understand that you are not unique in your victimhood, even though your circumstances might differ from that of others, it is much easier to let go of the emotions and feelings that allow you to begin having a loving happy life and eat just to nourish your body, not to feed your soul. It only took me about 60 years to realize that.

Disclaimer: *The following story is not so that you will feel sorry for me because that keeps me a victim. This story is to demonstrate that incidents from long ago can be a factor in your behaviour today.*

I was in an advanced Hypnosis course, it was near the end of the last day and again we had to partner up to practice a technique called the Timeline. It is a Hypnosis technique where you travel back along your timeline to the root of an issue while you are in trance.

My class partner and I completed the exercise even though we were tired and felt over saturated with information. My class partner went into Hypnosis first, we completed the technique and then it was my turn. I decided to do my weight as my issue and I could feel myself travelling back along the line. *Floating on my magic carpet, seeing the line below me...* When I touched down, I had a very strong feeling as if I were a newborn baby. As my class partner began to ask me questions, I thought that if I opened my mouth to answer, I would make a noise like a newborn crying. I clamped my mouth closed and didn't answer any of her questions. She brought me back to present time and emerged me. She felt she had not completed doing the technique with me. I quickly assured her that what she had done was very powerful. I then told her about feeling as if I were a newborn and what I suspected I had uncovered. I wasn't sure and told her I had to confirm it with my older sister and I really hoped my sister knew the answer.

My sister confirmed that my Father believed that if you "trained" the baby to sleep through the night, starting from the very first night after we came home from the hospital, then there would be none of that nonsense getting up all hours of the night. Calves on the farm were separated from the milking cows about a week after they were born, so why wouldn't it be the same for newborn children? So he would not let my Mother get up to us in the night and after crying it out, we just slept through the night. I connected the dots that when my Mother was first away from home – even though I was 12 or 13, that the **feeling inside** was that I wanted to eat and eat and eat. That is my first recollection of feeling deprived.

When I got married, I had three children very quickly. Those were the days when the Doctor only allowed you to gain 20 pounds during the entire pregnancy. That was when I began starving myself the day before my monthly Doctors appointment. I wanted to avoid the lecture and disapproval from the Doctor about gaining too much weight. I valued pleasing the Doctor more than the health of my own baby growing inside me. So my second experience with deprivation was the difficulty to keep to those 20 lbs the Doctor wanted me to do during pregnancy.

After each birth I went back to my original weight and was really quite thin. So thin at that point that my husband bought a product at the drug store called "**Wate ON**".

I googled it recently and there were several articles talking about it in the 1960's and later.

Here were the ingredients: (*not that we even read the labels* then)

> **Active Ingredients:** Per 2 Tablespoons (30 mL): Total Fat
> (Saturated Fat 2.5g) 15g; Sodium 10 mg; Total Carbohydrate
> (Sugar 2g) 5g; Vitamin A 2000 IU; Vitamin C 20 mg;
>
> Vitamin D 200 IU; Vitamin E 15 IU; Thiamin 0.75 mg;
> Riboflavin 0.51 mg; Niacin 10 mg; Vitamin B6 1 mg; Vitamin
> B12 3 mcg; Biotin 0.015 mg; Pantothenic Acid 5 mg; Iron 9
> mg; Zinc 7 mg; Copper 1 mg.

**Can you see from the above ingredients how low the grams are?
Sugar – 2 grams? I think my toothpaste today has 2 grams of
sugar.**

> **Inactive Ingredients:** Hydrogenated Stabilized Soybean Oil;
> Water; Sugar; Propylene Glycol; Polyoxyethylene 20 Sorbitan
> Monolaurate; Sorbitan Monostearate; Xanthan Gum; Methyl
> Paraben; Sorbic Acid; Artificial Flavoring; Propyl Paraben;
> Ferric Citrate; Niacinamide; Panthenol; Pyridoxine
> Hydrochloride; Riboflavin 5 Phosphate; Thiamin
> Hydrochloride; Calciferol; Vitamin A Palmitate; Ascorbic
> Acid; dl-Alpha Tocopherol Acetate; Biotin FFC; Copper
> Sulfate; Zinc Oxide; Artificial Color; Butylated
> Hydroxytoluene; Cyanocobalamin.

**(Yikes – What the heck are all those other ingredients and they
call them Inactive ingredients)**

I continued to be very thin once I had the babies and was caring for
three children under five. I believe that was the beginning of my mind
and body experiencing an unhealthy body image.

Body image is not related just to over weight but any criticism of your shape and size and the way you feel about how your body looks to yourself and what you perceive others see and think about your body parts.

It is important to love and accept yourself, including your physical body parts. If you love and accept yourself and your body, this journey becomes easier immediately.

In my forties, I was working at my daughters dance studio and left the house every day at 4:00 pm. I left my husband's dinner all made and ready to heat up but as the fast food establishments sprouted up on every corner, it was easier to buy something for myself and eat it at my desk. It certainly was economical and that is how I justified it to myself.

I hardly noticed when the pounds started creeping on. My height hid a lot of pounds and I seemed to gain it evenly all over. I went up a size; and then another and still was in complete denial. Once I passed size 16, I tried on an outfit I really liked but found I would have to go to size 18 to fit into it properly, I woke up with a jolt. All of a sudden, I saw fat everywhere on my body and in pictures of myself that I perceived I looked awful and I jumped on the diet train.

The puzzlement that my body would not co-operate with my complete deprivation was monumental. The failure I felt when for the first time in my life I was big. The denial about how I looked and the shock I felt when a picture or a mirror confirmed that I was overweight. The criticism I gave myself, the names I called myself when time after time the train would go OFF the tracks.

I just kept thinking it was the diet's fault. So every new book and diet that came out, every diet pill, every program on TV, every interview, and every grocery store magazine at the checkout became my study group.

Many of my clients relate that they have also done everything I have listed in the previous sentence. I now tell them that instead of this being a negative or a failure, they need to pat themselves on the back that they were that persistent and still are in still looking for the solution that works. Our determination actually helps to rule out what isn't helpful and keeping what did work and getting us to the point of finally finding a solution that will be with us forever.

One of the methods I tried was to join a popular weight chain that weighed you several times a week and gave you needles for the cravings and I lost 50 pounds. I instinctively knew the way I was eating was not healthy and was not going to be a lifelong way of eating. Once I lost the weight and stopped going to the program, I gained back the weight. Instead of feeling like a failure, I celebrated that I could now rule out unhealthy fad programs that have such a dramatic quick solution. I was still searching for the solution that could sustain and balance my weight for the rest of my life.

The Virtual Gastric Band and Exhale Weight Program is a long, slow process of losing perhaps one pound a week. If you were to be over 50 pounds lighter a year from now would that be wonderful?

Reality Shows, Human Nature and Weight

I love reality shows on Television. I find them a fascinating study in human nature.

I really feel that watching "The Biggest Loser" even though I didn't participate at home, just watched, was helpful in programming my mind to eventual success. Every book we read, every program followed, every presentation listened to, leads us in the direction of eventually getting a lifestyle change in place and feeling in control of our eating patterns.

"Survivor" taught me that you couldn't blame your height, family history, genes, DNA, body shape, thyroid, allergies, hypoglycemia, blood sugar etc. – Because –

EVERYONE on Survivor loses weight.

I had to face the facts that it is all about how much you put in, and how much you burn off – calories in and calories out. Portion size.

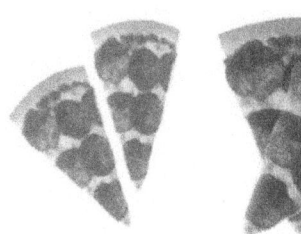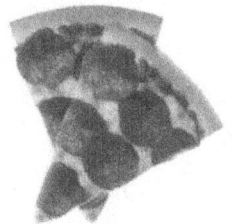

Food portions
20 years ago vs. Today

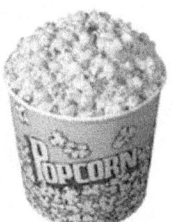

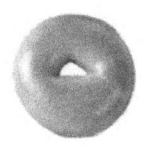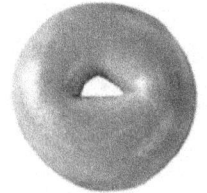

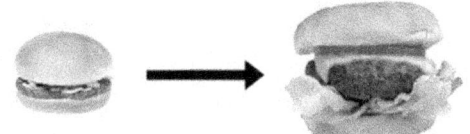

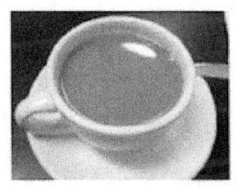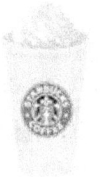

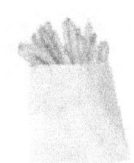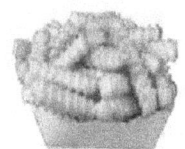

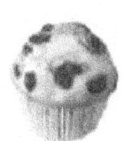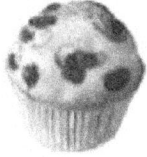

The life force energy and nutritional value of our food is also a factor.

We are eating food that is made and packed in foreign countries. We are eating produce, fruits and vegetables that are picked green and ripened unnaturally. Food that is filled with ingredients we know nothing about. We are eating GMO foods and not even aware of what they are and which foods they are in, or how our bodies process these changes.

We are eating processed, boxed or packaged, manufactured food that isn't real food. Real food is grown in the ground, picked from trees or plants, seeds, grains, animals or animal products such as meat, fish and eggs.

Leptin is a very important hormone that helps regulate appetite and metabolism. It is produced by fat cells, and sends a signal to the part of our brain that tells us to stop eating. The more fat contained in fat cells, the more leptin they produce. People with obesity produce very large amounts of leptin.

People with obesity could also have a condition called leptin resistance. So even though our bodies are producing leptin, it is possible the brain doesn't see or recognize it. When the brain doesn't receive the leptin signal, it wrongly thinks that it is starving, even if it has more than enough body fat stored. Some of the ingredients and preservatives in our foods today can also block the leptin signal.

Bottom Line: Leptin resistance is common in people with obesity. The brain doesn't sense the leptin that is produced, so it thinks that we are starving. This causes a powerful physiological drive to eat more.

Through the hypnosis part of the program, we remind the brain and the body to work together in always paying attention to that "I have had enough signal"

Clients report back how surprised they are to feel that full signal again. The Virtual Gastric Band with Hypnosis is a non-surgical lap band takes care of the physical controls and allows you to feel full at each and every meal.

You can override the band. The result of doing that is feeling overfull similar to eating that second helping at Thanksgiving or Christmas and then feeling too full.

I also have a personal believe that we can eat massive amounts of processed or snack foods because of the lack of nutrients in them. Clients have revealed that they can eat an entire bag of cookies or an entire bag of potato chips.

Why don't they feel full until after finishing so much?

Some report they don't even feel full after finishing. Is it possible that some of the chemicals or preservatives or ingredients in these products are blocking what should be our body's natural response when the stomach is full?

In the movies, when boy meets girl and everything is sunshine and roses and then they have a disagreement. Hollywood likes to show the girl in her pajama onesie, sobbing and eating an entire tub of ice cream with a big spoon. Making her look cute and vulnerable as she soothes her emotional experience. I have seen this over and over in many different movies or television shows. She is supposed to look cute and funny holding a big spoon and soothing herself with comfort food. How many people give themselves permission to soothe with food after seeing that example repeated over and over? Very subtle hypnosis suggestion, In action.

Food is not the enemy. We need food to sustain our bodies. We need to eat to nourish our bodies – not to soothe our soul.   When I took "Sheila Grangers" course on installing the Gastric Band with Hypnosis, I felt immediate hope and excitement that this could be the turning point for many people. When I came home from the course, another Hypnotist who had attended with me installed the band on me and I installed the band on him.   Years later, I can still feel my band working. I can still overeat and not listen to the full feeling but the result is that I feel overstuffed and uncomfortable. My stomach feels stretched and it is not a pleasant feeling and not a feeling that is repeated often.

It is more than the physical feeling though. I feel so in control when I eat my meal, feel full, and stop. I feel fully satisfied.

Emotional Eating: "It is what it is"

If you own a dog, do you ever notice that they can feel guilty, but never hold on to the emotion? My dog woke me up to go outside in the middle of the night. Then very early in the morning was whining to go out again. She had already thrown up on the carpet by the door and rushed by it with a guilty look. She came back in and went right to her cage because she knew I was upset with her as I scrubbed the carpet.

An hour later when my husband came down, she bounded over to me, the signal that it was breakfast time. She had a happy eager look on her face and I couldn't help but laugh.

Why do we as humans hold on to every emotion we can imagine?

Whatever we think that we have done or whatever has been done to us in the past – It is what it is.

No matter how big or small the incident is that has us feeling guilty, sad, depressed, angry, fearful, anxious – it is what it is.

We can't feel guilty enough to change the past - it is what it is.

We can't feel sad enough to change the past - it is what it is.

We can't feel depressed enough to change the past - it is what it is.

We can't feel angry enough to change the past - it is what it is.

We can't feel fearful enough to change the past - it is what it is.

We can't feel anxious enough to change the past - it is what it is.

Forgive yourself, move on, and let go.

It doesn't mean that you have blatant disregard for your actions – just don't waste your time on what you cannot change

"We are always in the moment in time we are supposed to be, therefore there are no shoulda, woulda, coulda's in my life"

If you should have, you would have. Going back and thinking of different ways you should, would or could have acted in any moment in time sets up "regrets". It is a way of thinking that has no value, purpose, or benefits to our well-being.

When I did a Thesaurus search for synonyms for the word regrets - here is the list:

Anguish apology, bitterness, concern, contrition, disappointment discomfort, self-accusation, self-condemnation, self, disgust, self reproach, woe, dissatisfaction, grief, heartache, heartbreak, misgiving, qualm, remorse, repentance, sorrow, uneasiness, worry, affliction, apologies, conscience, lamentation pang penitence scruples

When I did a search for Anonyms, here is the list:

Calmness, comfort, contentment, delight, happiness, joy, pleasure, relief, satisfaction, contentedness

We are all in the moment in time we are supposed to be.

A very wise lady told me this odd example probably 35 years ago. I thought it was very hard to figure out, and it kept popping into my mind every so often. As I look back over my life, it is absolutely true.

Imagine a room full of people. There are two men in the corner. One begins a violent fight with the other. Everyone has free will to decide the appropriate action to take in this situation. We can call 911, we can run out the door, we can hide, we can just stare, like a deer in headlights, we can jump in between them, we can hide, scream and yell or any other possibilities we can think of.

Whatever we all decide to do (many will be the same, many will be different) **and it all happens in a split second,** *we all end up in the exact moment in time we are supposed to be.*

The one man is supposed to dominate the other, the other man is supposed to be beaten; whatever each one of us decides to do is exactly what we are supposed to do. There are no shoulda, woulda, coulda's later. We cannot choose wrong. We are ALWAYS in the moment in time we are supposed to be. Regretting later that you should have done something different is generating a regret.

I found the concept to be unbelievable and arrogant – whatever we decide to do is always right. Whatever we decide is exactly what is supposed to happen – no responsibility for decisions.

As I look back on many decisions in my life, it is absolutely true.

Sometimes we <u>think</u> we made a wrong choice but it inevitably took us to where we needed to be.

Ho'oponopono Mantra

I have not studied Ho-oponopono and do not know the whole technique or how or why it works.

Whenever faced with a stressful, or irritating situation, if you just keep saying these words over and over.

The situation solves itself - usually in your favour.

It also works for when a phrase, an incident or a song keeps playing the tape over repeatedly in your mind. The moment it pops into your mind, say these phrases over and over.

It will stop popping into your mind.

"I'm sorry.

Please

Forgive Me.

Thank-you.

I Love You."

Jo-Anne's Ten Commandments

1) When we try and stop our latest eating program, instead of beating ourselves up, and feel like a failure, why don't we pat ourselves on the back and congratulate ourselves for at least trying. Congratulate yourself that you made it for one day, one week, or one month. Celebrate that you tried. Celebrate that you are aware. Celebrate that you care about yourself. Celebrate your success!

2) I AM PERFECT WHOLE AND COMPLETE EXACTLY AS I AM IN EACH   AND EVERY MOMENT IN TIME!

3) I love and accept myself 100%. I love and accept everything about myself. I am a good person.

4) I am always in the moment in time I am supposed to be in.

5) I am completely aware at all times about my self-talk. At no time do I call myself names, for any reason or about any situation.

6) There are no mistakes in my life and no "shoulda, woulda coulda"

7) If it doesn't get done today – Oh well!!!!!

8) I love my life, I love my circumstances, I love my family, I love where I live, I love my car, I love my work, I love my job, I love my friends and I love my dog. I am thankful and grateful.

9) I am not defined in life by anything other than love. I live in the heart, I breathe from my heart, I act from my heart.

10) There is no person, thought, idea, memory, image, feeling or sensation out of the past, in the present, or ever to arrive in the future that could change me from feeling inwardly happy, peaceful and fulfilled.

Part Two:

Revitalize Your System

"Whatever I choose,
is ALWAYS right for me."

The Candida Cleanse

Fungal yeast overgrowth in the human body is not taught in medical schools. So despite the fact that autopsies have found kidneys and other organs literally clogged with yeast cells most doctors have not had any training in fungal yeast overgrowth and often deny that it even exists.

When I realized that for the first time in my life, I couldn't lose weight just by cutting down and being more active, I went to see a Holistic Practitioner who explained yeast build up in the body to me. When I first heard this information, it made total sense to me.

We all have a certain amount of yeast in our bodies and if we gorge on too many carbohydrates and foods high in sugar, it builds up in our body and causes us to continuously crave <u>more</u> carbohydrates and sugar.

I went home with the following Yeast or Candida Cleanse (below) and Monday morning, 7:00 am, I started, eager and determined. I kept the paper in front of me and followed it to the letter.

By 10:00 o'clock I had a slight headache and my nose was running a little. I thought to myself that I must be coming down with something.

By lunchtime, my head was throbbing and my nose now was running continuously and I thought I had a full-blown cold. I phoned the practitioners office to ask if I should continue the cleanse while I had a cold.

It was explained to me that I did NOT have a cold but rather my body was already responding to the cleanse, and that the headache was caffeine withdrawal and the runny nose was sugar withdrawal and the yeast was already dying off in my body and that I was doing very well. It was called a "Healing Crisis"

By the end of the day I felt like I had a full blown flu and that a truck had run over me - several times - and that I did not like this Candida Cleanse at all.

The next morning, I did not feel very much better. I am very stubborn and somewhere in my fuzzy brain and aching body was knowledge that if it felt this bad getting yeast out of my body, then it shouldn't be there and this was a good thing.

I expected that the worst was behind me. HA HA HA HA HA!

By the end of the second day, I felt even worse and wondered if something else was going on, so again I phoned the practitioner and told her I was dying. I wasn't any better; in fact I was 10 times worse. **Exaggeration** did not work on her at all, but she did say I could have some forbidden beets for supper, which might ease the symptoms because beets have natural sugar in them.

I had beets for supper along with a few other permitted foods and she was correct. In a few hours the symptoms eased a little.

The next morning as I urinated and then turned to flush, to my horror the toilet was filled with a bright pinks bordering on red. Again, I panicked, emergency phone call to my health practitioner, positive I was bleeding from the kidneys and bladder. She laughed and asked me if I had eaten the beets the night before. Mystery solved, and no, I wasn't bleeding from the kidneys and bladder.

Another day of misery as the pesky flu like symptoms persisted, although not as bad as before. I cheated again that night eating a forbidden sweet potato for the sugar.

Thursday morning dawned bright and cheery and so did I

I felt great! Cravings were gone and there was a sense that I had done something wonderful for my organs and my body.

I have since learned to <u>gradually eliminate</u> coffee and foods ahead of time to avoid the healing crisis.

<u>Candida Cleanse Definite No – No's:</u>
Remove COMPLETELY from your diet.

1. No Bread
2. No Potatoes
3. No grains
4. No dairy
5. No Fruit

<u>Avoid the Following:</u>

- Sugar and sugar containing foods. Sugar and quick acting carbohydrates including sucrose, fructose, maltose, lactose, glycogen, glucose, sorbitol, galactose, monosaccharide, and polysaccharide.

- Also avoid honey, molasses, maple syrup or other sugars.

- Yeast, Breads and Pastries - Raised baked goods, including breads, rolls, cakes and pastries containing bakers yeast.

- Alcoholic Beverages - Avoid all of them.

- Condiments, Sauces and Vinegar containing foods - Mustard, tomato sauce, Worcestershire sauce, soya sauce, pickles, olives, horseradish, fruit mince and tamari. **Also avoid sprouts.** Vinegar of all kinds and vinegar containing foods, such as mayonnaise and salad dressing.

Freshly squeezed lemon juice may be substituted.

AVOID THE FOLLOWING

- Processed and Smoked Meats - Pickled and smoked meats and fish including sausages, hot dogs, corned beef, bacon and ham.

- Dried and Candied Fruits - Raisins, apricots, dates, prunes, figs, apples, pineapples and papaya

- Left-over's - Moulds grow on left-over food unless it is promptly and properly refrigerated

- Fruit Juices - Either canned or bottled or frozen including orange juice, grape juice, apple juice or any other fruit.

- Coffee and Tea - Regular coffee and teas of all sorts **including herb tea**

- Melons - Watermelons, honeydew melons and especially cantaloupe

- Edible Fungi - All types of Mushrooms

The Candida Diet:

✓ Foods Allowed

Artichoke	Asparagus	Beetroot
Beans (green)	Broccoli	Brussels Sprouts
Cabbage	Cauliflower	Celery
Chokos	Corn	Cucumber
Carrots	Eggplant	Lettuce
Marrow	Onion	Pumpkin
Peas	Parsnip	Radish
Sweet Potato	Spinach	Turnips
Tomato	Zucchini	Peppers

✓ Drinks:

- **WATER ONLY** (can add a squeeze of lemon)
- **Freshly made vegetable juice** (carrot and celery)

✓ Allowed All Proteins

Beef	Chicken	Crabs
Duck	Eggs	Fresh Fish
Lamb	Lobster	Oysters
Prawns	Rabbit	Salmon
Tuna	Turkey	

✓ Raw Nuts:

Almonds	Cashews	Pecans
Pine Nuts	Pumpkin Seeds	Sesame Seeds
Sunflower Seeds		

✓ OIL: 2 Tablespoons Daily

- Avocado Oil
- Butter
- Sesame Oil
- Sunflower Oil
- Cold Pressed Olive Oil

The Sugar Factor

Humans have relied on a remarkable, naturally occurring hormone called leptin to regulate what we ate, **and it told our brains when we'd had enough**. But somehow in recent years that regulator has become confused, and suddenly it seems like people just don't know how to stop eating because the signals that tell your body you're full seem to be no longer working.

Too much sugar over stimulates your brain's pleasure center, leading to addiction.

And if you pull back on the substance, you go into withdrawal. Tolerance and withdrawal constitute addiction. It is now being reported by several experts that **sugar is addictive!** If you have withdrawal from a substance when you completely stop ingesting it, the body system craves it. Alcohol, nicotine, drugs, and sugar.

Sugar is pleasing in the moment when it passes through your lips, the more you eat the more you crave – and ultimately the more you'll *need* to eat to get those same pleasurable feelings. This sugar addiction can actually re-wire your brain. Of all the molecules capable of inflicting damage in your body, sugar molecules are probably the most damaging.

Fructose, in particular, is an extremely potent pro-inflammatory agent, and speeds up aging.

It is perfectly normal for your blood sugar levels to rise slightly after every meal, it is not natural or healthy when your blood sugar levels become excessively elevated and stay that way - which is what will happen if you're eating like the typical North American, who consumes on average a staggering 2.5 pounds of sugar a week! Other low-quality carbohydrate-rich foods such as white bread, sugar, donuts, pasta, pastries, cookies, and candy, also break down to sugar (starch is broken down into glucose) in your body and often contain *added sugar* as well. It's not so difficult to see why so many North American people carry excess weight and are in such poor health.

Cancer cells thrive in an acid environment. It is difficult to lose weight when the acid/alkaline is not in balance. A diet made of 80% fresh vegetables and vegetable juice, whole grains, seeds, nuts and fruits help put the body into an alkaline environment. About 20% can be from cooked food including beans. Fresh vegetable juices provide live enzymes that are easily absorbed and reach down to cellular levels within 15 minutes to nourish and enhance growth of healthy cells.

To obtain live enzymes for building healthy cells try and drink fresh vegetable juice (most vegetables including bean sprouts) and eat some raw vegetables 2 or 3 times a day. Enzymes are destroyed at temperatures of 104 degrees F (40 degrees C).

The Five Worst Foods for Your Body

Excerpt from "The Five Absolute Worst Foods You Can Eat"

by Dr. Mercola   (www.mercola.com)

Doughnuts:

Doughnuts are fried, full of sugar and white flour and most all varieties contain trans fat. Store-bought doughnuts are made up of about 35 percent to 40 percent trans fat, and an average doughnut contains about 200 to 300 calories, mostly from sugar, and no other nutrients. It is dough. NOT ONE NUTRIENT

Trans fats, found largely in commercially prepared baked and fried foods, have become notorious in recent years because they not only raise harmful LDL cholesterol, but also lower levels of heart-healthy HDL cholesterol. High trans-fat intake has been linked to coronary heart disease, in which fatty plaques build up in the heart arteries. When foods are cooked at high temperatures, carcinogenic substances like acrylamide can form.

People view doughnuts as a breakfast food when there are so many other positive choices to break fast and nourish our bodies. Nutritionally speaking, eating a doughnut is one of the least effective ways to start off your day. It will spike your blood sugar and doesn't provide any real nutrients. Eating a sugary carbohydrate food, results in soon being hungry again.

Soda:

One can of soda has about 10 teaspoons of sugar, typically in the form of high fructose corn syrup, 150 calories, 30 to 55 mg of caffeine, and is loaded with artificial food colors and sulphites. I can't think of any good reason to ever drink it.

The diet varieties are even less beneficial as they are filled with harmful artificial sweeteners like aspartame and/or sucralose.

Studies have linked soda to osteoporosis, obesity, tooth decay and heart disease, yet an estimated 50 gallons of soft drinks are consumed each year. Drinking all that sugar will likely suppress your appetite for healthy foods, which pave the way for nutrient deficiencies.

A 20-ounce glass of cola contains the equivalent of 16 teaspoons of sugar in the form of high fructose corn syrup (HFCS). This is nearly *three times the maximum daily sugar intake* recommended by the American Heart Association. HFCS typically contains a mixture of 45 percent glucose and 55 percent fructose (although recent investigations have found that many brand-name sodas actually contain *65 percent fructose!*).

Once ingested, your pancreas rapidly begins to create insulin in response to the sugar. The rise in blood sugar is quite rapid.

Here's a play-by-play of what happens in your body upon drinking a can of soda:

- **Within 20 minutes,** your blood sugar spikes, and your liver respond to the resulting insulin burst by turning massive amounts of sugar into fat.

- **Within 40 minutes,** caffeine absorption is complete; your pupils dilate, your blood pressure rises, and your liver dumps *more sugar* into your bloodstream.

- Blood glucose level 79 at the outset of the experiment, and after 40 minutes it had risen to 111.

- **Around 45 minutes**, your body increases dopamine production, which stimulates the pleasure centers of your brain – a physically identical response to that of heroin, by the way.

- **After 60 minutes,** you'll start to have a blood sugar crash, and you may be tempted to reach for another sweet snack or beverage.

Chronically elevated insulin levels (which you would definitely have if you regularly drink soda) and the subsequent insulin resistance is a foundational factor of most chronic disease, from diabetes to cancer.

Lately, the media has finally begun reporting on the science of fructose, which clearly shows it is far worse than other sugars. Fructose is processed in your liver, and unlike other sugars, most of it gets shuttled into fat storage. This is why fructose is a *primary culprit* behind obesity—far more so than other sugars.

According to the news report above, drinking two bottles of soda per day can make you gain a pound of fat per week! If you routinely drink soda--regular or diet--**eliminating it from your diet is one of the simplest and most profound health improvements you can make.**

Fried Food: Anything that is fried, even vegetables, has the issue of trans fat and the potent cancer causing substance – acrylamide.

Foods that are fried in vegetable oils like canola, soybean, safflower, corn, and other seed and nut oils are particularly problematic. These polyunsaturated fats easily become rancid when exposed to oxygen and produce large amounts of damaging free radicals in the body. They are also very susceptible to heat-induced damage from cooking. What is not commonly known is that these oils can actually cause aging, clotting, inflammation, cancer and weight gain.

You can google the article "Secrets of the Edible Oil Industry" for more information.

It is theoretically possible to create a healthier French fry if you cook it in a healthy fat like virgin coconut oil. Due to its high saturated fat content, coconut oil is extremely stable and is not damaged by the high temperatures of cooking.

This is why coconut oil is an excellent choice to use and cook with.

One French fry is worse for your health than one cigarette, so you may want to consider this before you order your next "Biggie" or "Supersize" order.

Chips:

Most commercial chips, and this includes: corn chips, potato chips, tortilla chips, and dorito chips, are high in trans-fat. Fortunately, some companies have caught on to the recent media blitz about the dangers of trans-fat and have started to produce chips without trans-fat.

However, the high temperatures used to cook them will potentially cause the formation of carcinogenic substances like acrylamide, and this risk remains even if the trans-fat is removed.

Fried Non-Fish Seafood:

This category represents the culmination of non-healthy aspects of food. Fried shrimp, clams, oysters; lobsters and so on have all the issues of trans-fat and acrylamide mentioned above, plus an added risk of mercury.

Seafood is loaded with toxic mercury and shellfish like shrimp and lobsters can be contaminated with parasites and resistant viruses that may not even be killed with high heat. These creatures, considered scavenger or bottom feeder fish consume foods that may be harmful for you.

to be free of harmful levels of mercury and other contaminants – the delicious wild red Alaskan Salmon.

Complete Lifestyle Change

The biggest change in the way we think about releasing weight is that this program is NOT a diet. My clients continue to think or state that foods are forbidden or "bad" to eat

Diets are Boring - You Need Constant Willpower and Discipline

It is impossible to stay focused and motivated ALL the time, and that causes "slipping" or "falling off the wagon" and the dreaded F word - Failing

Diets Are Really Easy to Fail At

Most diets require you follow the plan to the letter all the time. When you slip it is really hard to start again and really easy to keep slipping.

Your Mind Thinks of Diets as Temporary

Usually diets are seen as a change in behaviour until a certain amount of weight is lost, but what happens then?

Diets Eventually Make You Feel Deprived

Diets focus on what you can't eat, and that naturally increases, the feelings of missing out on something.

A lifestyle change for the remainder of your life to maintain a healthy desired weight where you eat three small meals a day, stop when you are full, no snacking in between.

You have just finished a section on the 5 worst foods you can ingest by Dr. Mercola. If this isn't a diet, why can't I have those foods? The good news is you can. You can eat anything you want, as long as it is within your three meals a day, stop when you are full and no snacking in between meals.

The difference is that once you begin to release the weight and begin having more energy, feeling more positive, and actually enjoying this new way of eating, your brain makes a switch and you begin looking at foods in a different way.

When clients come in and tell me they have had a bad week, or a bad day where they ate foods they know they shouldn't have – (their words NOT mine.) I quickly point out to them that there are no bad foods or good foods and that they can have anything they want, stop when they are full and no snacking in between. If you have had a day where you ate something out of the ordinary, well - good for you. We all love a treat now and then. Just for that time, the food was in control and now you are back in control because you recognize that. Now let's look at what is eating you that day that allowed the food to be in control.

Once people learn and fully comprehend that food doesn't solve problems for them, those times when you feel like gorging on everything in sight are few.

I like to introduce the concept that foods are not good and bad. Foods are high vibration and low vibration foods and there is a difference. By changing the way we talk about and label food, it gives it a different importance in our lives.

My dowsing group did an experiment where they measured five foods for two categories - life force energy and nutritional value, each out of 100. One of the items of food was an organic apple that measured very low in both categories. My dowsers were sure their calculations were wrong until I told them it was an organic apple from New Zealand. It very well could have been picked green, ripened unnaturally, travelled by train, truck, boat, and plane and probably sat in warehouses along the way before it arrived in the store. So their dowsing indeed was correct.

Then we placed three of the items of food on or in three various devices made to raise the vibration of the food items. We also dowsed with our pendulums with the intention to raise the vibration over one food and we said a prayer over the final item.

The result of our experiment was that every method actually worked and did raise the Life Force Energy of the food and also the Nutritional Value of the food. The method that raised it the highest percentage was prayer. A simple grace said over the food made it more beneficial for our bodies.

Table Prayer
I bless this food before me.
I honour this food for providing me sustenance.
I send blessings to everyone who participated in the growing or preparation of the food.
I send my love and light to all those in need.
I send my love to mother earth
And I send love to the creator of our universe.
And so it is,
AMEN

Part Three:

The Exhale Weight Program

"Every morning say to yourself: Something wonderful is going to happen to me today!"

About the VGB and Exhale Weight Program:

This program is a combination of the Virtual Gastric Band (VGB) with Hypnosis technique that works on the physical aspects of releasing weight.

Exhale Weight is an outstanding and effective holistic approach to life-long weight management and understanding the emotional factors to provide the solutions you are seeking.

A New Approach to Weight Management

1) The Exhale Weight Program addresses the emotional components while the VGB non-surgical lap band takes care of the physical aspects and allows you to feel full at each and every meal.

2) Really understand the relationship that food has in your life and begin to eat - just to nourish your body - not to soothe your soul.

3) Techniques to use that make it so easy to manage your own self-sabotage when it comes to food.

In Summary:

The **Virtual Gastric Band with Hypnosis Program** utilizes a non-surgical technique that allows you the ability to feel full when eating.

The Exhale Weight program addresses the **emotional**

aspects of releasing weight and the **relationship** we have with our food.

What is the Virtual Gastric Band and How Does it Work?

The Virtual Gastric Band is a non-surgical technique, developed by Sheila Granger from the UK, for Hypnotists worldwide to use the power of hypnosis to retrain your mind and body to work together and be satisfied with smaller portions of food. It changes how you think about food and gives very safe, very predictable results. You can eat what you want, during your three small meals a day. The Virtual Gastric Band will enable you to intake smaller portions. This can be your long-term solution to finding success with weight and your relationship with food. Many clients worldwide have benefited from The Virtual Gastric Band technique.

Benefits of the Virtual Gastric Band Method:

- No Complications of Undergoing Invasive Surgery
- It's Cost Effective
- A Clinical Trial proved **95% Successful**
- A Cutting Edge Technique for Modern Weight Solutions
- **This new lifestyle is simple and easy. Three meals a day in which you eat what you want,stop when you are full, no snacking in between.**
- No dieting, no depriving yourself.

The Entire Program consists of four Sessions:

Session 1: Introductory Session

Initial session where the Virtual Gastric Band with Hypnosis is 'installed'. Learn how you can incorporate the Exhale Weight program into your life to make lasting changes and take control of your weight and your relationship with food. Are you ready to change your life?

Session 2: One Week Later

Scheduled one week later and can be as short as one hour or as long as 2 hours, depending on how well you have done and what ideas have surfaced for you. Each and every client is different in his or her approach and previous experience

Session 3: Scheduled within the month.

It is scheduled usually within a month –Stretching out the time for you to see how easy it is to continue on your own. I am always a phone call or email away if you need me for any situation that arises. Many things can be briefly addressed over the phone.

Session 4: Follow-Up

Can be taken at any time - from just after Session 3 or even months later. If you need some help in new ways; your weight has plateaued, for various reasons; or you have strayed off the program and want to get back on track; or just to tell me and show me how well you are doing.

Personal One-on-One Session

May be required after initial program is complete. It is up to the individual to book their own sessions when needed.

Eight Golden Rules for Success, of the Virtual Gastric Band Procedure:

© Sheila Granger | Lifestyle Engineering Limited – 2012

Make a resolve now to take responsibility and follow these simple rules and success will be yours.

1. Buy Something New

One very powerful psychological technique is called the law of concentrated attention. It means that if there is something in life that you really want – then behave in a way that you already have it – and you are very likely to get it.

Buy an item of clothing one size smaller than you currently wear. It can be as simple as a T-shirt or a full outfit. Hang that item of clothing where you will see it first thing when you wake up and frequently at other times of the day. Seeing your new item of clothing reinforces in the mind that it is yours and it fits. When the item of clothing is physically there, it will be accepted in the mind and in the present moment.

2. LISTEN TO THE SUPPORT CD – DAILY

The CD utilizes a multitude of the latest mind management and is important that you listen at least once a day for the next 28 days. The CD will create new neural pathways in your brain regarding your associations and attitudes towards food. It will also reinforce the live sessions that you attend. You will increase the effect tenfold if you listen to it using stereo headphones via your iPod or a CD Walkman, or computer

3. EAT SLOWLY AND CONSCIOUSLY

Enjoy every mouthful of food, slow down, chew your food thoroughly and enjoy the flavours and textures. Put your knife and fork down between mouthfuls if necessary. Digestion begins in the mouth. Do not eat in front of the television or while reading, as you will not be as conscious of what you are eating. Sit down and focus purely on the food in front of you. Thoroughly enjoy your food. Food is there to nourish your body, not to soothe your soul.

4. STOP EATING AS SOON AS YOU FEEL COMFORTABLE

Leave the remainder on the plate. There is no need to finish once you feel full. After some time has passed this exercise of leaving food when you are full will leave you feeling very in control.

5. EAT ONLY THREE SMALL MEALS A DAY

As your portion size will be dramatically reduced, it may be worth investing in some smaller plates and bowls.

6. BUY AND TAKE SOME GOOD QUALITY VITAMINS.

7. DRINK PLENTY OF FLUIDS AND CHOOSE ONLY LOW CALORIE LIQUIDS

Water can be flavoured with Essential Oils. Herbal Teas, Coffee – 2 cups per day. Black Tea – 2 cups per day. Grapefruit juice. Tomato Juice – read label. *Soda Pop whether regular or low calorie or sugar free and pasteurized juice from the store are very high in sugar content. Choose wisely.*

8. EXERCISE

It is beneficial with the gastric band that you take up some form of exercise for 30 minutes per day. This can be as simple as going for a walk.

If you already belong to a gym and attend, then continue enjoying your membership. If going to the gym has never been part of your life then it is not likely that you will go faithfully if you were to join. Some gyms have several free visits to attend before making the decision to join. Try it out. Perhaps you will love it and it will become part of your life. There are some gyms that have a pay as you go plan. That might be a better choice if you are not sure you will go months from now.

If you already are certain that a gym membership is not something you want to do, then find other ways to move and use your body that you would enjoy. Joining a gym and then not going is costly to your finances and also your feelings of success. Success is what we strive for in all aspects of this program.

I run up the stairs in my house. There are 15 steps. At first I was winded and breathing heavy but now years later it is easy.

When I am out, I take the stairs whenever I can rather than the elevator or escalator. If I take an escalator, I step up the steps even though they are moving unless someone is in the way. I park farther away from the doors of anywhere I am going and walk briskly into the store or business.

Exercise will communicate to your body that you want to use your muscles and force it to burn the fat. Walk, skip, and dance around the house – MOVE AND HAVE FUN!

Lymphatic System

The **lymphatic system** is a network of thin vessels that branch, like blood vessels, into tissues throughout the body. It is part of the immune **system**. It is a one-way **system** which carries cells and fluid back to the blood **system**.

A pale fluid that contains white blood cells and that passes through channels in the body and helps to keep bodily tissues healthy

There are extensive explanations and websites if you want to know more about this. Take a closer look at the important role your **lymphatic system** plays in keeping your body balanced and **healthy**

As with every system of the body, if it is tuned up and working properly, the benefits to your health and weight are obvious.

Getting sluggish lymphatic systems and organs flowing smoothly is the key to easy weight loss and improved feelings of well-being. If you are suffering from injuries, excess weight or cellulite, or pain disorders like arthritis, bursitis, headaches, a sluggish lymphatic system may be playing a role.

One of the ways to keep the Lymphatic system draining and healthy is rebounding on a mini trampoline, which can dramatically improve lymph flow and it also gets your heart rate up so you get exercise in easily. Begin jumping 100 times and gradually increase what you can do.

What is Hypnosis?

Hypnosis is a state of focused attention and heightened suggestibility. There are many other explanations, some of them quite lengthy but none explain it as well as those few words.

Excerpts from the "National Guild of Hypnotists Learning Manual":

"Hypnosis refers to a state or condition in which the client becomes highly responsive to suggestions. The hypnotized individual seems to follow instructions in an uncritical, automatic fashion and attends closely only to those aspects of the environment made relevant by the hypnotist.

Hypnosis is considered to be a unique and separate state of consciousness, relative to one's "normal" state of consciousness. In this concept, the trance is a state that is created by the trance induction process. It alters the person's consciousness through the narrowing of attention to the offered suggestions."

Myths about Hypnosis:

"The hypnotist will be in control of me"

Hypnosis properly done, you are always in complete control of your Session. Your hypnotist is just a guide.

"I may reveal all my secrets"

Hypnosis is not a truth serum. You will only share with your hypnotist what you are willing to share.

"You might get stuck in Hypnosis"

Contrary to recent news articles, you cannot get stuck in Hypnosis.

Without constant dialogue, Hypnosis cannot be sustained.

Subjects in Hypnosis would emerge themselves.

Jo-Anne Eadie is a Certified Member of the National Guild of Hypnotists.

Summary of Jo-Anne Eadie's qualifications in Hypnosis

- Board Certified Master Consulting Hypnotist
- NGH Certified Instructor of Hypnosis
- Practitioner of Sheila Granger's Virtual Gastric Band with Hypnosis Technique.
- Licenced, Certified Trainer for the Sheila Granger Virtual Gastric Band with Hypnosis
- Past Life Regression
- Pain Management Certification
- Spirit and Entity Release
- Rapid Induction and Stage Hypnosis
- Counselling Skills with Hypnosis
- Hypnosis for Childbirth
- NLP Basic Practitioner
- Sports Psychology with Hypnosis
- Super Success with Weight Solutions
- Certified 5PATH Hypnosis Practitioner
- The Simpson Protocol
- Smoking Cessation Specialist

Part Four:
Understanding a New Approach

"I trust and I know."

Weight Loss Sabotage

Have you had this experience? You look in the mirror and start to think, "I feel good. I look great."

You're dropping the pounds. The extra exercise is paying off. You're fitting into clothes that haven't fit for years.

You're just starting to think you finally are on the right track. Old habits and beliefs begin running the program and the self talk says:

> *I will have to maintain it.*
>
> *You keep losing weight and your sister will feel bad!*
>
> *You keep losing weight and your husband will be jealous.*
>
> *Your whole family is fat; if I get skinny they'll judge me.*

That old fear, anxiety, sadness, or grief comes crashing in on you. Then the pangs of guilt and shame flood back in and it's off to the refrigerator for some something tasty.

Thus the cycle of binge-shame-eat-again starts all over...and over...and over. All your promises, best efforts, and good intentions crumble as the old program of soothing with food begins anew.

If your focus is only on changing your outer world circumstances and that is all you put your attention on, you will likely get more of the same.

This is basic Law of Attraction – what you focus on expands.

As strange as it sounds, you must:

Put your attention on changing your inner world and how you feel about your outer circumstances.

If you can come to a place of peace concerning that, then your outer circumstances will change. Feel good within yourself and the outer world will change to match how you feel. Let that be the ONLY thing that matters.

If you want your life to change, you must change it first from the inside. Then the outside will align with that.

Think about this for a moment: *How do you feel on the inside right now when you think about your outside life?* That is what is being projected outside to your life.

Change the inside and the outside must change and align. Focus only on the outside and get more of the same.

Why we eat so much:

We have lost the ability to feel full and we have been programmed to accept larger portions as normal. When I was taking Sheila Granger's Virtual Gastric Band course, it brought back a lot of memories.

I remember that I never took anything for recess to school. No one ate anything at recess. We went out to play.

We only ate three meals a day and I don't remember anyone in the kitchen after we did the dishes from our evening meal. I can really feel that full feeling part way through my meal and now realize that I have not felt that feeling for quite a few years and that I have been eating too large of a portion at a meal.

Why do we eat more than we are supposed to?

We rely on a remarkable, naturally occurring hormone called leptin to regulate what we eat, and it told our brains when we'd had enough. But somehow in recent years that regulator has become confused, and suddenly it seems like people just don't know how to stop eating.

I believe that today's food are so void of nutrients and life force energy that we are starving to death even though so many people in North America weigh far more than is healthy.

We eat foods that are out of season from where we live. The foods are picked green, shipped by plane and boat and truck and trains and stored in warehouses along the journey and ripened by artificial means.

It is just a theory on my part that we can eat and eat and eat because the foods that we eat are not nutrient dense, and therefore just pass on through never really nourishing or feeding our body.

In my Hypnosis practice, it is common that clients don't feel good enough about themselves. When using EFT – Emotional Freedom Technique, the opening statement states what we are working on and ends with "I deeply love and accept myself" People will often tap on it but when asked if they do love and accept themselves, people will tell me honestly that they don't. Some will tell me they hate themselves. We work on loving and liking ourselves just the way we are right now. This is a big piece of the puzzle of figuring out their weight.

I Walk Down The Street – Portia Nelson

Chapter One

> **I walk down the street.**
> **There is a deep hole in the sidewalk. I fall in.**
> **I am lost... I am helpless.**
> **It isn't my fault.**
> **It takes forever to find a way out.**

Chapter Two

> **I walk down the same street.**
> **There is a deep hole in the sidewalk.**
> **I pretend I don't see it. I fall in again.**
> **I can't believe I am in the same place.**
> **But, it isn't my fault.**
> **It still takes me a long time to get out.**

Chapter Three

> I walk down the same street.
> There is a deep hole in the sidewalk.
> I see it is there. I still fall in. It's a habit.
> My eyes are open. I know where I am.
> It is my fault. I get out immediately.

Chapter Four

I walk down the same street.
There is a deep hole in the sidewalk.
I walk around it.

Chapter Five - I walk down another street."

Understanding Your Relationship with Food

Bring your awareness to how you feel / respond to the following:

- o I eat when I'm happy
- o I eat when I'm sad
- o I eat when I'm bored
- o I eat when I'm upset
- o I eat when I'm angry
- o I eat when I'm lonely
- o I eat when I'm hungry
- o I eat when I'm not hungry

I eat when I'm _____

I eat or drink too much:

- candy
- cookies
- dessert
- donuts
- muffins
- cake
- chocolate bars
- chocolate
- potato (chips with or without dip)
- peanuts
- doritos
- french fries
- french fries with gravy
- is poutine
- bread
- fully loaded baked potato
- mashed potatoes and gravy
- melted butter on just about anything
- Nachos
- FAST FOOD
- beer and wine

- I think that I eat too large of a portion
- I think that I take second helpings
- I think that I eat the wrong kind of food
- I think that I binge on certain foods at times
- I think that I snack in between meals
- I think that once I nibble and snack, I can't stop
- I think that I don't seem to know when I'm full
- I think about food a lot. I watch the clock and feel thrilled when it is mealtime.

- o I talk a lot about food. I like to tell people about good restaurants and the selection on the menu and their appetizers, entrees and desserts. I like to describe what I had and how good it was and I like to hear a description about what they ordered and how they liked it.

- o Eating out is a major source of enjoyment and the largest part of my social life.
- o A large buffet with many different items from appetizer to dessert is: _____

- o I think that I just really like food

- o I like the food in my mouth, chewing and swallowing and taking the next bite. I'm disappointed when I am finished my meal or snack.

When I have binged or overeaten, I

- o I hate myself
- o I feel sad or depressed
- o I call myself names
- o I feel like a failure
- o I swear I will never do that again
- o I cry

While I'm overeating, I say things like:
- o I know better.
- o One more won't hurt
- o I've been good all week
- o I eat healthy most of the time
- o I will exercise extra hard to wear this off
- o I might as well eat the whole think and get it out of the way.

Control

There are many people, myself included, who for various reasons do NOT like to be told what to do. They don't like their husband or wife coworkers or Boss to tell them what to do and will vigorously protest if that happens.

We don't like the feeling of government telling us what to do. We don't allow friends to tell us what to do and certainly won't let someone we don't like to tell us what to do.

And yet:

- Food controls us 100% Food is the BOSS
- Food can be very persuasive when we are feeling emotions that we don't like.
- Food beckons and wins every time.
- Food tells us what to do no matter how hard we try.
- Food is in charge of most of our day.
- Food sneaks up on us and we mindlessly finish large quantities and then are surprised that we did that.
- Food proves we have no will power over it. We try to say NO and we are successful – sometimes, but in the end, food is the more powerful force.
- Food is repetitive. No matter how many times we have tasted something, we want it again.

Who is in charge?   Who is in control?   Food.

Being Controlled   Controlling Others   Controlling Situations

I don't think anyone likes to be controlled. Even if you think you don't think you mind being controlled, it is human nature and perfectly understandable when finally one day the thought comes that:

"I've had enough!"   *"Leave Me Alone"*

Most people eventually react to control with anger. We may shout at a spouse or boss or parent or friend:

"Stop trying to control me"

We live in a fast food service world, a drive through banking world, an instant gratification world, never get a live person, press one, press two, world. It is becoming more and more common that standing in line, waiting for service, can't find a sales person, not being able to speak to a live person until you have gone through 15 minutes of voice commands. All of it and more makes us feel **controlled, manipulated, bossed around, anxious, angry and also hopeless and beaten down.**

WOW – I don't consciously feel that way. I think I manage my life pretty competently. It sounds and feels like truth that I do feel that way. It has a familiar ring of truth to it.

We give in and don't resist because there is nothing we can do about it. It wears us down and eventually we just give up and give in and reach for something we think will soothe us.

Subconsciously, we are still upset. Many times we will have a reaction that has nothing to do with the situation we are in, and everything to do with the constant frustration of being controlled. As much as we protest that we hate this or don't like that or why do they have to do it that way, we feel that we have no choice and realize that it isn't going to go our way.

Stress is the result of insisting that things be other than the way they are.

Now that we have uncovered and realized that we don't like being controlled, but we are controlled in so many ways in our lives, why do we allow food to be the boss? Why do we let food control our finances, our thoughts, our day, and our feelings?

Men and women begin the day, preparing breakfast for family, making lunches for themselves and their children and asking themselves "what will we have for dinner?" Do I need to go to the grocery store?

The thoughts and actions of feeding family members and our selves invade our life and so many snack items have become so accessible.

Coffee shops and fast food restaurants springing up everywhere making feeding ourselves so much easier to manage. The consequences of these visits go on the back burner as the convenience in this busy world take over.

If the pre-planning isn't done, the fast food industry fills the gap.

Why do we schedule our lives around food? Why do we jump through hoops for food? Food is one area in our life that we DO have total control over and yet we live our lives the opposite way around.

NOT TRUE – YOU SAY

Top Ten Ways Food Controls Us:

10. We can be tempted and we can overeat bypassing any logic or common sense, stuffing ourselves over and over. We wouldn't think of spreading a whole bottle of moisturizer on ourselves. We wouldn't wear three sets of clothes, layering one after the other. We wouldn't take 15 tissues to blow our nose once.

9. We will pay any price for an item of food or beverage – if we want it. The coffee shops come to mind where a single cookie is $1.25 or more.

8. We will knowingly eat products that have ingredients that are harmful to our health. Additives, preservatives and ingredients we cannot pronounce.

7. We will find a way to override any logic if we think it tastes good and we like it. Yes…I know but...

6. We will finish our children's food if they don't finish it.

5. We will call ourselves names, berate ourselves, and feel shame because of what we eat. We would be angry if someone else did this.

4. Even when we swear we will never overeat again, deep down we know we will and we do. How many people have had a really bad hangover? We swear we will never do that again – and we don't.

3. If a large bag of potato chips is on the counter, as long as it is not opened, I will NEVER touch it. If someone else opens it, I can't leave it alone until it is gone. I begin with just one small bowl, then another...and one more...and...oh well, I haven't had chips in a long time. If I finish them, they won't tempt me anymore.

2. We feel completely wasteful if we go to an all you can eat event/restaurant and just have one plate. We feel deprived if we only have one plate. We feel silly sitting there if we only have one plate and the others are going back for more. We feel left out, tempted, we have an inner struggle, should I get some more? Will someone notice if I get more?

We justify and make it a sensible choice to go get more. They are only going to throw it out if it is left there.

THE # 1 REASON WE KNOW FOOD CONTROLS US IS:

1. We will stand in line, or sit in our cars inching forward to get coffee and doughnut or bagel or breakfast sandwich.
No matter how long it takes!

- We will wait behind annoying people who are buying for 14 other people
- People or toddlers who don't know or can't decide what they want.
- People who are long lost friends with the cashier.
- Seniors who pay for one small coffee with a credit card to get the air mile points and can't remember there pin number.
- We don't complain or walk out because the coffee shop is the friendly place everyone goes to be happy
  And because the food and beverage industry own us.

We are controlled by them!

"I am in total control of what I eat, when I eat and how much I eat!"

Copy this Quote, make it as big as the page, and have it displayed: by your computer –by your bed –in your kitchen –one by your television and anywhere else you will see it regularly.

Intermittent Fasting

If you want to burn fat, intermittent fasting is a pretty good way to do it. Intermittent fasting is the time in between your three meals. This is a good reason to stick to your three small meals a day.

This is another reason why eating six small meals a day or three meals and three snacks is NOT your best plan.

It benefits the food industry but not you!

They know that telling someone whose eating is already out of control to eat more often, will result in them eating more and their profits going up. Eventually we tell ourselves that we are doing something beneficial by kick-starting the metabolism. What usually happens is that many expand those small meals and snacks to larger portions.

Normally, after a meal, there is a period of time where you're burning blood sugar [glucose] and then liver sugars [liver fat] or [glycogen], which are the carbohydrates stored in your liver and other tissues but particularly in the liver from your last meal.

It takes several hours for your body to fully digest your breakfast. After that you start to shift to burning fat. If you then eat again at 10:30am your body stops burning fat and again returns to digestion.

Your body ends up in perpetual digestion.

After a fast, even a short one you are burning body fat - normal and safe. Again between lunch and dinner, you are fasting and the body has a chance to burn off stored fat.

If your portion of food is too big from the last meal, there is un-used blood sugar in your system. Your body will preferentially burn blood sugar first delaying the job to burn fat.

If the blood sugar is used up before the next meal, the body robs the stored body fat from its hiding places. Body fat now flows around in the blood and is used to power the body, and slimming you down.

Exercise speeds up burning both blood sugar and fat. If you are exercising in a fasting state, like in the morning, before breakfast, or mid-morning, you will be burning fat, faster, easier, and more effectively.

Eat dinner, stop when you are full, not to eat afterwards until the morning. When the digestion is complete and the blood sugar is gone. now your body burns fat. You are burning fat while you are sleeping. Even the time between breakfast and lunch - lunch and dinner it is more beneficial for your body and your weight loss to allow your body to fast. Now it is just another exciting reason to let go of snacking in-between meals.

In addition, through the night when you are resting, your organs an all other body systems can rest also.

If you stay up until midnight and you are eating – healthy OR unhealthy snacks, new blood sugar is generated, and the existing blood sugar is never used up and the fat stores are never used up.

By the time you wake up in the morning, you still have in blood sugar your body and your body has not had a chance to burn any body fat at all. Now the surplus blood sugar tells your body to make more fat.

Your body needs to rest along with you after digesting your dinner meal all night until BREAK   FAST

Define Success

This is a long slow method of eating lifestyle – a program for the rest of your life. If you lose one pound per week, and this time next year you are 52 pounds lighter – is that success?

If the body image exercise helps you to change the way you think about yourself and your body parts to loving and accepting your body and youself – is that success?

If you begin thinking about the situation before reaching for food when you feel emotions of any kind that you previously thought soothed your soul – is that success?

When you know that the only job for food to do is to nourish your body - is that success?

If you really understand the concept of "Who is in Control?" and it permeates into all of the different facets of your life – is that success?

If embracing the concept of "Who is in Control?" allows you to experience personal power over food and the way you think and eat – is that a success?

If losing weight becomes secondary in your thoughts and just living in the present and enjoying life moment by moment - can you count that a success?

If you have released the need to lose weight, your mind and body become congruent and success begins to happen.
If you no longer obsess about food and now that you are aware, you also realize that you didn't know that you obsessed about food – is that a success?

If you no longer are obsessed with losing weight and you hardly think about it, enjoy your food and because of that you are releasing weight, is that a success?

If food is bossing you around, beckoning you and winning, it is likely that the loss of personal power is present in other relationships and areas of your life – not just food. Perhaps you are a people pleaser and you need to put yourself first.

Will every client lose weight? There isn't a program out there that has 100% success measured in pounds. During the four or more sessions, all of the above concepts are so simple that clients often don't notice and attribute their success to the different way they are thinking and eating.

If a client walks out of my door feeling better than when they walked in, I am fulfilled.
Is that success?

Part Five:
Exhale Weight
Mental Exercises

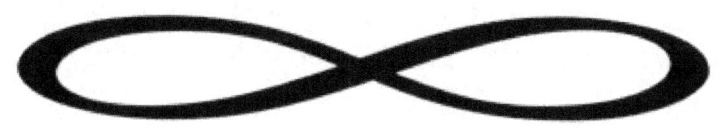

To avoid criticism:

Say Nothing
Do Nothing
Be Nothing"

-Aristotle

<u>Exercise 1:</u>   **Daily Tapping Routine**

Everyone gets up in the morning and brushes their teeth. Some floss and some also use mouthwash. Whatever your tooth brushing routine is, add this daily tapping routine as part of your tooth brushing protocol.

If you haven't done your daily tapping, it will therefore mean that you have not brushed your teeth that day.

- ❖ Tap on the beginning of the eyebrow at the bridge of the nose and say: *May I be free of suffering.*
- ❖ Tap at the side of the eye where the arm of glasses would go and say: *May I know the joy of my own true nature.*
- ❖ Tap under the eye (also a good point for nausea) and say: *May I be happy.*
- ❖ Tap under the nose on the upper lip and say: *May I be at peace.*
- ❖ Tap on the chin in the groove between the lip and bottom of chin and say: *I am an unlimited, strong courageous free spirit.*
- ❖ Tap on the collarbones, the bones that surround the hole in your neck where you swallow and say: *I accept all the blessings of life.*
- ❖ Tap on the top of your head and say: *I am thankful and grateful for all that I have.*

Paste the list (below) on your bathroom mirror once you have memorized the points.

It will remind you to **brush your teeth, floss and then tap**.

May I be free of suffering
May I know the joy of my own true nature
May I be happy
May I be at peace
I am an unlimited, strong, courageous free spirit
I accept all the blessings of life.
I am thankful and grateful for all that I have

If you do this for 30 days, it is guaranteed to change your life as many of my clients have attested. Many people end up doing it multiple times a day but I just require it once in the morning – minimum.

Take the challenge and prove me wrong!
Email me with your results, whatever they may be -
joanne@poweroffreedom.ca

Anger Dissolving

One of the problems with anger is that it often causes us to automatically react to the situation. These automatic anger reactions are almost never helpful and usually once you get angry – you lose.

A rapid routine for displacing anger, this method will both dissipate anger and help you choose a more appropriate response.

When you sense yourself becoming angry: Tell yourself you are going to allow yourself to be good and angry for five minutes.

During those five minutes while you think about how angry you are:

- Take a long, slow, deep breath.

- As you exhale slowly, visualize your anger escaping with your exhalation of air.

- Where do you feel the anger in your body? Insert a tube to allow it to escape. Is your tube large or small, plastic or rubber or something else?

- The anger will escape. Is it smoke? Liquid? Something else? Is it leaking out? Gushing out? Pulsing Out?

You'll be happily surprised at how well this works.

Ho'oponopono **Mantra**

I have not studied Ho-oponopono and do not know the whole technique or how or why it works.

Whenever faced with a stressful, or irritating situation, if you just keep saying these words over and over, the situation solves itself - usually in your favour.

It also works for when something negative keeps playing the tape over and over and over in your mind. The moment it pops into your mind, say these phrases. It will stop popping into your mind.

"I'm sorry.

Please

Forgive Me.

Thank-you.

I Love You."

Exercise # 2

30 Seconds Every Night for the next 3-Weeks

This exercise utilizes the power of the subconscious mind quite effortlessly, and gets people used to feeling good and builds up confidence levels with very little effort and time involved.

There is an epidemic of people not feeling good about themselves. Subconsciously, every television commercial we have watched since childhood has told us we are not good enough. Example: Our hair is not shiny enough unless we use this brand of shampoo.

We look at ourselves in the mirror or a picture and mentally judge and criticize what we see. We find fault with ourselves and at times are our own worst critic. We speak to ourselves in a critical and insulting way - a way we would never do with others.

We are all born perfect, whole and complete and that is the way we stay, and that is the way we are. Are there things we want to change or improve? Yes, maybe, but there is nothing wrong with us just as we are.

Body image is important and acceptance of yourself NOW is the key. If you don't like yourself NOW – you will find things wrong with yourself when you are thin.

The body you currently have may be out of shape and perhaps there are bulges where you would prefer them not to be. This is your present reality. If you ignore it or deny it or hide it, most of all from yourself, you increase your stress levels, grind your confidence into the ground, and set up all sorts of biochemical sabotage mechanisms. And in the morning, your body reality is the same as it was yesterday.

Here are the Rules:

Do it every night, without fail, for a minimum of three weeks, better for a month. Do not change the rules or add or subtract what you do – no more and no less.

Before you go to bed, look into a full-length mirror with all your clothes off.

Look at your body beginning at your head and as your eyes go down your body, say these words: release judgement. As your eyes come back up your body, say: release criticism

Turn one quarter turn so you can see one side of your body in the mirror and Look at your body beginning at your head and as your eyes go down your body, say these words: release judgement. As your eyes come back up your body, say: release criticism

Turn one quarter again and scan over your shoulder or with a hand held mirror and Look at your body beginning at your head and as your eyes go down your body, say these words: release judgement. As your eyes come back up your body, say: release criticism.

Then to the final side and scan up and down and finally back to the front - final scan up and down each time saying –
release judgment, release criticism so that your mind cannot form a negative thought. So you cannot say anything to yourself.

Finish by looking deeply into your own eyes for about 10 seconds, increasing it as you go along and tell yourself "I love you" "I am perfect just the way I am."

That's it – 30 seconds every night for three weeks.

Digestion Exercise

From the newsletter – chetday.com

A technique from Dr. Stanley Bass

If you need assistance with digestion, experience sequential eating,

This technique works beautifully for a lot of different people
Here's what you need to do to eat sequentially:
Instead of eating beans and then potatoes and then salmon, eat all of
one food first and then go on to the next item on your plate.

For this to work suitably, you need to eat the least dense food first and
the most dense last.

If your dinner consists of salad, green beans, boiled red potatoes, and
salmon.

To practice sequential eating, you'd eat all of each item in this order:

- Eat all the salad.
- Eat all the green beans.
- Eat all the potatoes.
- Eat all the salmon.

Give it a try for a week and see your results.
What have you got to lose?

Part Six:

Exhale Weight Program Techniques

"I am not defined in life by anything other than love. I live in the heart, I breathe from my heart, I act from my heart

EFT Tapping Points for the Basic Recipe

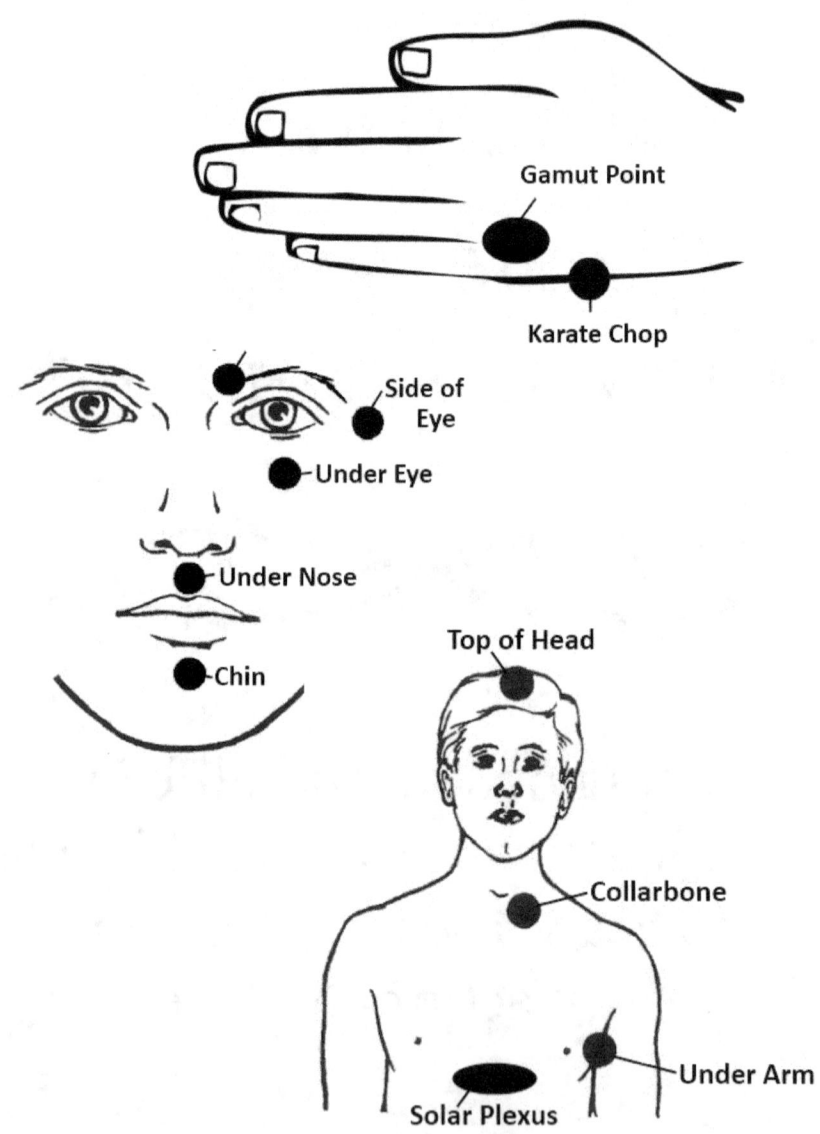

The Basic Recipe

A very forgiving technique, it does not have to be perfect to work

Set Up Affirmation – Using three finger tips on the Karate Chop and say:

"Even though I have _____I deeply and completely love and accept myself.
(Example – Even though I have a headache) Say this sentence three times

Move to the following points saying small reminder phrases on each point. To keep you focused.

Tip of the eyebrow
Side of the Eye
Below the Eye
Upper lip
Chin
Collar Bones
Under the breast across the ribs (anger points)
Under the arm
Top of the Head

Continue With:

Tip of the Thumb
Tip of the Index Finger
Tip of the Third Finger
Tip of the Baby Finger
Karate Chop
Gamit Spot – Top of the hand between the ring finger and the baby finger

Additional EFT Statements for the Basic Recipe:

Tap on the points saying:

Even though I am scared I will feel deprived

Even if I don't lose one pound on this program

Even if no other program has ever worked for me

Even if I think this program will not work for me

Even if I want a snack after dinner, I choose to not eat anything after 7:00 pm

Even if I weigh _____ I choose to weigh my normal weight which is _____

My normal weight is_____ (affirmation) and that is what I weigh

Even if I don't like the way I look in the mirror, I choose to love & accept myself exactly as I am.

Even if others don't like the way I look, I choose for that to be their problem, not mine.

Even if I want that cookie now, I choose to have it later.

Even though I am scared I will feel deprived

Even if no other program has ever worked for me

Even if I think this program will not work for me

Even if I want a snack after dinner, I choose to not eat anything after 7:00 pm

Tap on these statements over and over:

It is only natural that I have this feeling, but I'm ready to let this go.

I deserve to be free of this and I'm ready to let this go.

There is no reason to keep this, and I'm ready to let this go.

It is safe to release the weight easily and freely

I am ready to let go

I deserve to let go

I need to let go

It's safe to let go

I want to let go

It's easy to let go

It is possible to let go

Psychological Reversal Corrections

A psychological Reversal is when you want to lose weight, but the mind and body are not on the same page. Example: You want to release weight an you do but you no longer fit in with your friends who are still overweight. You will sabotage your own success trying to subconsciously please them.

Say these affirmations three times while tapping the karate chop (fleshy side of the hand where Karate experts would use to break a board.

Or say these affirmations while **rubbing the sore spot). draw a line from mid shoulder down to and with your other hand over from the armpit across. That is where the lymph sore spot is.**

Affirmations

I deeply and profoundly accept myself with all my problems and limitations

I deeply and profoundly accept myself even though I have this problem.

I deeply and profoundly accept myself even though I still have some of this problem

I deeply accept myself even if I never get over this problem.

I deeply accept myself even if I deserve to have this problem.

I deeply accept myself even if I don't deserve to have this problem.

I deeply accept myself even if it is not safe for me to be over this problem.

I deeply accept myself even if it is not safe for me to be completely over this problem

I deeply accept myself even if it is impossible for me to get over this problem.

I deeply accept myself even if it is impossible for me to completely get over this problem

I deeply accept myself even if I am ashamed, embarrassed or humiliated getting over this problem

I deeply accept myself even if I am blamed or criticized if I get over this problem.

I deeply accept myself even if I am blamed or criticized if I completely get over this problem.

I deeply accept myself even if I won't survive if I give up this problem.

I deeply accept myself even if I will be disloyal to my Mom/Dad/Aunt/ Uncle/Cousin/Friend/Boss/Co-Worker if I let go of this problem.

I want to let go of this problem
I need to let go of this problem
I deserve to let go of this problem
It's time to let go of this problem.
It's safe to let go of this problem
I'm ready to let go of this problem

"A Gratitude Experiment..." by Carol Look

What if we assumed that everything the Universe sent to us was "good" for us...even if we didn't see it that way at first?

That would mean that everything that happened during our day was something positive, even if we had a negative reaction or interpreted it as "bad" initially.

This new assumption would certainly change our energy quickly, wouldn't it?

Many people routinely expect bad things to happen, and when their beliefs are fulfilled, their reaction is *"Well, that's typical for my life..."* or *"I knew it wasn't going to work out..."* or *"Same old...same old..."*

So if we started with the assumption that absolutely ***everything*** that showed up in our lives was potentially positive and offered a special opportunity, then we'd be expressing our gratitude by saying *"Thank you, Universe"* all day long... hmmm... I wonder what that would do to our vibration if we were saying "thank you" that often.

I guess we won't know until we conduct an "experiment." Here is what I am proposing: **(I'm not saying it will be easy, I am just extending an invitation...)**

Set your intention for the next 24 hours (start whenever is best for you) to interpret every experience, person, phone call, email, social or business interaction that comes into your life as something potentially wonderful, something that has hidden magic, as something that is a beautiful gift even if it shows up in lousy wrapping paper. And several times an hour, after each short time period in your day or after each interaction, say ***"Thank you, Universe for bringing that*** *into my life... I'm so excited and looking forward to understanding why it is so positive for me."*

OK, I can hear the "**Yes, but**" reactions right now!!! Did you have any of these following reactions?

This is so corny.
This doesn't feel "normal."
But bad things always happen every day - they're just bad, why would I be grateful for them?
I don't feel grateful on a good day, so why bother?
I'm sure this won't work for me.
I don't get the point anyway!

That's fine if you have any of these reactions, and you don't even need to accept my invitation to try this new experiment. That's up to you -- try it or not.

But I want you to understand why I am proposing the experiment before you decide whether it is for you or not. What's the "point" of this experiment? Ultimately, to raise your vibration which will help get you on the fast track to attracting abundance. Here are several essential points to this experiment:

(1) To shake up the old energy patterns you've been running.
(2) To deliberately move your expectations from pessimistic to optimistic.
(3) To raise your vibration.
(4) To consciously be in contact with the habit of thanking others.
(5) To consider the possibility that everything that shows up IS good, even when it doesn't seem that way at first.
(6) To communicate to the Universe that you are interested in things that delight you and that you want more of them.

One of my favourite expressions that has helped me slow down my initial impulsive and negative reactions to situations that don't feel good is:

More will be revealed...

And I have come to believe and experience that there is always more to be revealed in any situation. Here are some suggestions of how you might ease yourself into saying "thank you" to the Universe even if you don't really feel like conducting this "experiment."

Hmmm, something that looks and feels lousy just happened, but it's possible that I don't know all the energy around it... so I guess it's possible it might turn out to be a good thing after all. Thank you, Universe.

That's fascinating; yet another annoying person just crossed my path... I wonder if there's a good reason and I just can't see it yet. I'm willing to withhold my judgment and my reaction until I get more information. Thank you, Universe.

Interesting... that project didn't go as I thought it would, and now I'm feeling irritated and disappointed. I wonder how I can turn this around. Maybe I can tap first, and then thank the Universe for sending me something that I trust will turn out well in the end. Thank you, Universe.

When you express genuine appreciation for what's in your life, you will notice dramatic new levels of energetic support from the Universe.

So what might get in the way of your not being able to thank the Universe for everything that comes into your life?

(1) You expect things to go wrong.

(2) You are a perpetual cynic.

(3) You prefer to expect the worst from people and from life.

(4) You feel safer when you are down... this way you can't get surprised.

So even if you have some "good reasons" not to try this experiment, you might want to try it just for fun... or just to see if it changes your vibration... or in case it does work to raise your vibration quickly... or just because it's super simple or to prove that it doesn't work

> *Thank you Universe for everything you sent me today,*
> *I know that more will be revealed about those*
> *challenges I don't understand yet...*

So no matter how "good" or "bad" something seems to you today (and this week) make the assumption that it is good, that it will yield wonderful results, that it may look bad now, but you will soon be able to see its purpose and place in your life.

> *You will raise your vibration as soon*
> *as you decide to focus on basic*
> *appreciation to the Universe*
> *for everything that happens*
> *in your life.*

As you've heard from me and other *Law of Attraction* teachers before -- *it's all energy*! Moving from one genuine statement of thanks to the next will invite the Universe to help you create more abundance today.

Remember, the *Law of Attraction* sends you situations that have the same energy of the vibration you are putting out... so keep thanking the Universe and emit that vibration of gratitude.

Below you will find **EFT/ Meridian Tapping** setup phrases to help you release the resistance to gratitude.

When you change your vibration,
you will change your life.

1. EFT SETUP PHRASES:
The **EFT SETUP Phrases** for this topic are as follows:

While tapping the **karate chop spot** on either hand, repeat these phrases out loud, (or change the words to fit your exact situation).

"Even though I don't feel very grateful for what went wrong today, I choose to accept myself anyway."

"Even though I don't feel like saying "thank you" to anyone for anything, I accept who I am."

"Even though it's not easy to be thankful for everything, I accept myself and how I feel."

I have indicated where to tap while saying each of the phrases below. You may repeat the positive round more than once if you wish. (Those of you who are new to **EFT** may view a chart of the spots on my web site under the EFT pages.)

Now for the phrases that focus on the problem

Eyebrow: *"I don't feel thankful today."*
Side of Eye: *"I only feel grateful for good things."*
Under Eye: *"I'm not sure I'm ready to change my viewpoint."*
Nose: *"I don't feel very thankful for what I think went wrong."*
Chin: *"Maybe I just feel like being upset."*
Collarbone: *"These upsetting feelings are so strong and valid."*
Under Arm: *"Why should I be grateful for everything?"*
Head: *"It's hard enough to get through the day..."*

Now for the positive focus on the solution

Eyebrow: *"What if I could try this new experiment?"*
Side of Eye: *"I can do anything for a day."*
Under Eye: *"I could try thanking the Universe for everything."*
Nose: *"I want to want to be grateful for everything that happens."*
Chin: *"I love feeling grateful, even for things that don't look that good to me!"*
Collarbone: *"I appreciate the Universe's messages."*
Under Arm: *"I love knowing the Universe is taking care of me."*
Head: *"I love feeling grateful for everything that happened today."*

Access more positive vibrations with the **Law of Attraction** *by repeating the following phrases (while tapping or not):*

Thank You, Universe for helping me feel genuinely grateful for everything you sent me today.
Thank You, Universe for allowing me to feel gratitude all day long.
Thank You, Universe for helping me to feel grateful for surprising events that showed up in my life.

Weight Releasing Tips, and Tricks

One of the tricks when you feel like snacking is to go and brush your teeth.

This accomplishes three things:

Once you have brushed your teeth, the minty taste makes you **feel** as if you have eaten something. Once you brush your teeth, you don't want to spoil a fresh mouth. Things don't always taste good right after you brush your teeth as it mixes with the minty fresh taste.

I grew up eating three meals a day. No one ate snacks at recess at school. We went out to play at recess. I can't remember anyone in our kitchen after dinner. It has become a "habit" to eat at coffee break or any other time other than meals spurred on by the food and beverage industry. Foods loaded with sugar, sweeteners and msg.

- Put a straw in a glass of water and sip it instead of gulping it. Sometimes it is just the arm motion to the mouth that is the habit.

When I am outside gardening I lose track of time and often even forget to have lunch until about 1:30 pm. Everyone can think of a time when they were very busy and worked right through a meal without feeling hungry.

When you want to snack - over analyze why you want to eat: Are you truly hungry? What is the emotion you are feeling right now? What emotion did you feel 10 minutes ago? What do you truly want? Are you thirsty? The craving is history, as your mind gets busy.

Inhaling certain aromas can actually help reduce cravings.

I inhale pure organic essential Young Living Oils such as Peppermint, Orange, Lemon, grapefruit, spearmint etc. A drop in a glass of water flavours it and is very satisfying. The oils are good for you and can help to cleanse.

Some foods, like fruit, are simple carbohydrates that are easily absorbed and result in a quick rise in blood sugar and energy. Fruit also has the benefit of containing water, fibre, vitamins and minerals. But if you add some low-fat or lean protein to your fruit, you can provide a steady stream of energy for several hours. Keep your portions small so you get the energy boost without the calories.

Your Serotonin levels may drop due to decreased carbohydrate intake. This can often be relieved by as little as 200 mcg of cooked spinach or a glass of fresh squeezed orange juice.

Don't use special occasions to break your pattern. If it is a birthday, think of the cake as part of your dinner - part of your meal.

Imagine...

- Every day when you are in the shower, as the water flows over you from head to toe – imagine it, see it, feel it, the pounds melting off with the water.

- If you soak in a bath, imagine it, see it, feel it, the pounds soaking off and going down the drain.

- Visualize and projecting images are very powerful tools.

NLP Spinning Technique

Hunger Pangs or Cravings

Close your eyes and locate where in your body the **craving** resides.

On a scale of 1 – 10, with 10 being the highest what is the number of the **craving**? Whatever pops into your mind is the right answer.

It may or may not have the following:
Does it have a shape?
Does it have a color?
Does it have a name?

If it were a spinning wheel, which way is it spinning? Clockwise or Counter clockwise? Or another way?

Bring it up and out in front of you

What is the shape now? If it is the same – change it.
What is the color now? If it is the same – change it.
Does it have a name now?
What way is it spinning now? If it is the same – change it.

Put it back into your body and note the number now from 1 - 10.
Repeat if necessary

Can be used for cravings, fears, anxiety, anger

Process to Wipe Out Fear utilizing the NLP Spinning Technique:

Choose a strong fear that you get in a particular situation, which holds you back in life (you should get scared just by thinking of it).

Feel the fear, at least a little. Instead of running away from this fear as you may usually do, let yourself actually feel it. Don't indulge in the fear, but just feel it enough to do the next step.
Notice where the feeling starts. As you feel that fear in your body, notice where it starts and where it moves.
(it may begin in your stomach and move up toward your chest and/or throat).

Imagine pushing the feeling out of you and seeing it spin as if it's a wheel in front of you. Notice, does it spin forward or backward? Clockwise or counter clock wise? If for some reason you're not sure which way it's spinning, just guess, as people almost always guess correctly. Also, if you're not able to visualize easily, just move your finger in the direction it is spinning.

If you're able to visualize, you can even add a color to the fear as you watch it spin around. If you cannot see it like a little tv in your head, you may be auditory or kinaesthetic. Sense, or imagine the fear. Either notice the color it already has, or give it a color you think is appropriate for the feeling of fear. (a lot of people choose red, for example). If you can't visualize this, imagine what it might be.

Turn the wheel upside down, so it's now spinning in the opposite direction. As you do this, if it had a color before, notice that now the color has changed to the opposite of fear (e.g., a calming blue or white).

Pull this new feeling back inside you so it moves in the reverse direction to the old fear (i.e., down from throat or chest, towards your stomach). Make sure you keep spinning this new feeling in the new direction.

As you spin your new feeling faster and faster, think of the same thing that scared you before. And, as you do this, you'll probably notice that you feel quite differently now about what you used to fear.

Now, get out there and make things happen in your life!

Hypnosis today has new techniques and new ways of dealing with problems without needing to re-experience the issues. On this new path, you find new ways to let go with Hypnosis of the things that keep us stuck and it becomes an easier and more pleasant experience.

Tip: Self Hypnosis is usually taught within the Hypnosis session. Here is the first step of Self Hypnosis. Tonight when you go to bed, lay on your back with your arms by your sides. Take a long slow deep breath in, and exhale with a sigh the experience of your day. Say to yourself "Every day in every way, I just get better and better" and lift one of your 10 fingers to keep count." Say it again "Every day in every way, I just get better and better" and lift another finger until you have done it 10 times and then allow yourself to gently drift off to sleep.

Eating Healthy

Eating healthy is a process that is gradual. It is difficult to just change over years of eating one way to complete vegan or vegetarian, or completely raw no matter how big the benefits are. Your taste buds switch over gradually as well. I have now begun to try to incorporate at least one raw dish into each meal.

Your taste buds need to gradually get used to eating differently.

Once you make the change, you can enjoy healthy items just as much as store bought treats loaded with sugar and preservatives your body doesn't even recognize.

I began by purchasing an industrial blender and making green smoothies. Apples and pears blended with Kale and spinach. Delicious. Adding cinnamon lowers your blood pressure. Ginger makes it tasty with a little spice. I have not included a lot of recipes in this book because you can find almost any recipe you want by using Google. Simply Google green smoothies and a multitude of websites and newsletters and recipes are at your disposal

Salad every day with more variety of ingredients makes them even more delicious. I add two tablespoons or more of hemp hearts and kale sprinkles and make salads even tastier. I love texture in my food so that really works for me.

We live on a farm and raise our own grass fed beef. When people eat our beef for the first time, they are astounded at the taste and puzzled why grocery store beef is so different.

Our Beef Cattle are Hormone Free, Grain Free and vaccine free. They graze outdoors in a pasture. During the winter months they are fed high quality hay. My husband is very picky about the Hay and never feeds mouldy hay or hay with bird droppings.

Our farm is clean and a beautiful environment for our animals.
Children on the farm pet them and use them in their 4-H projects showing them at the fair.
We use a small local butcher not a large slaughterhouse. The cows are humanely treated and housed.
Our animals are blessed and thanked for doing the wonderful job of being our food.
The meat is delicious and nourishing for our entire family and extended family, and all who eat this meat.
I believe that the way animals are treated and raised makes a difference in the quality of the meat making it tender and nourishing.

We also raise our own chickens that live outside and scratch around and eat clover and grasses and bugs and worms. We have planted fruit trees and have raspberry bushes and strawberry and blueberry plants. My husband grows a large garden and I can and freeze tomatoes and peaches and pears.

Many of our habits and beliefs are lifelong

There is a story about a young wife who cuts the eah end of the roast off and then puts it into the pan. One day, her husband asks her why she does this? Her answer is that is the way her Mother does it. So she asks her Mother why and her answer is that is the way Grandma did it. So they ask Grandma and she said her pot was too small and so she cut the ends off so it would fit.

Eat your crusts and you will grow big and strong.

I liked crusts when I was a kid but I had siblings that didn't and often heard the sentence about eating your crusts because they were good for you.

I told my children the same thing. My grandchildren were a different story. One day our youngest grandchild was over and asked for a peanut butter sandwich and could I please cut off the crusts. Of course I did. Grandma's break all the rules and let them do whatever.

While I was cutting off the crusts, I was thinking about how the sentence has been told to countless numbers of children and yet it isn't true. **The vitamins and minerals and goodness do not run to the outsides of the bread at any time of preparation and baking.** I had never thought it out before. I am still chuckling about that. It is more about waste than the crusts being good for you.

The food industry has us running in circles with all their advice. Their agenda is that they want to sell products and have nothing to do with them looking out for our health.

The following is an explanation that you can use to tell people some more important reasons NOT to eat in between meals. I have found with my groups that they have been so convinced to "graze" all day. A lot of "experts" in the field recommend 3 meals plus 3 snacks or six small meals a day. We are asking people who are having a hard time controlling their intake of food to eat more meals a day. We have found the following explanation helpful and beneficial for people who are tempted in between meals to have a snack. When they think of it as "fasting" in between meals and realize they are doing something very good for their body, it is easier to resist.

Eating Out at Restaurants

I LOVE to go out to dinner. I have been married for over 50 years I am just tired of making dinner daily. It is not a job you get to retire from. While I am a good cook, and an even better baker, I don't just love to make dinner. It is easy to order carefully when I go out and make good choices that allow me to go out often.

When you first change your diet no matter how gradual, you can end up constipated. It is surprising how the carbs and the sweets with no nutrient value can push through and keep you regular. I found that probiotics and enzymes added to my daily regiment, and the many glasses of water make those wrists to elbow floaters that your Naturopath delights in.

Enzymes are the most important ingredients for digestion and cooked foods have very little enzymes left. Anything pasteurized has all the nutrients boiled out of it. Probiotics and enzymes give you have great digestive health and elimination.

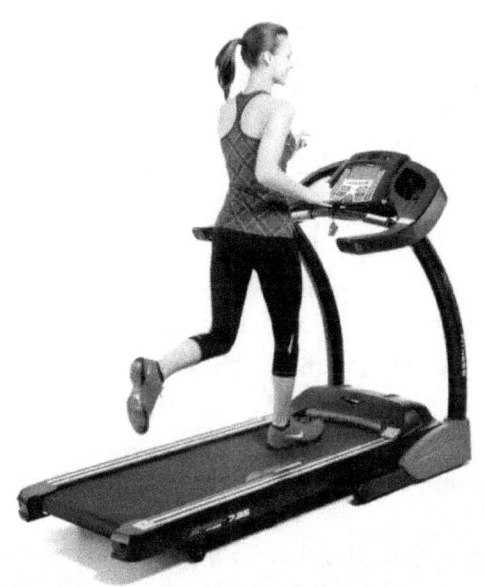

One hour on the treadmill burns 150 calories

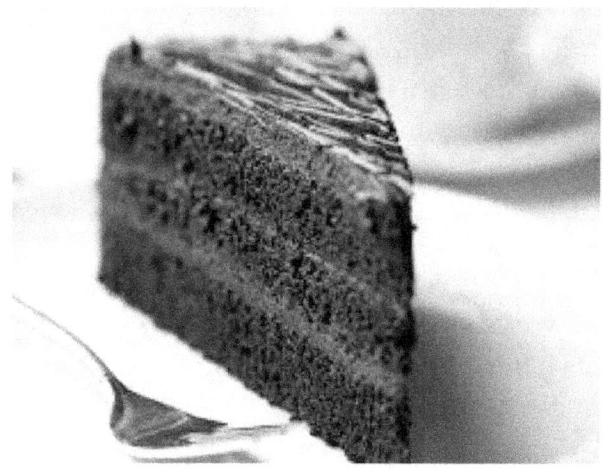

That piece of chocolate cake - 400 calories

Amazing frozen lemons:

All it is...is a frozen lemon!

Place the washed lemon in the freezer section of your refrigerator. Once the lemon is frozen, get your grater, and shred the whole lemon (no need to peel it) and sprinkle it on top of your foods.

Sprinkle it to your vegetable salad, ice cream, soup, cereals, noodles, spaghetti sauce, rice, sushi, fish dishes, whisky, wine, even in instant cup noodles... the list is endless. All of the foods will unexpectedly have a wonderful taste, something that you may have never tasted before.

Most likely, you only think of lemon juice and vitamin C.

What's the major advantage of using the whole lemon other than preventing waste and adding new taste to your dishes?

Well, you see lemon peels contain as much as 5 to 10 times more vitamins than the lemon juice itself. From now on, by following this simple procedure of freezing the whole lemon, then grating it on top of your dishes, you can consume all of those nutrients and get even healthier.

It's also good that lemon peels are health rejuvenators in eradicating toxic elements in the body.

So place your washed lemon in your freezer, and then grate it on your meal every day. It is a key to make your foods tastier and you get to live healthier and longer!

Your whole body will love you for it!

Paleo Bread

Ingredients

1 cup Quinoa Flour
1 cup blanched Almond Flour
2 tbsp coconut flour
1/4 cup ground golden flax meal
1/4 tsp celtic sea salt
1/2 tsp baking soda
4 eggs
1 tbsp liquid coconut oil
1 tbsp liquid honey
1 tbsp apple cider vinegar
1/2 tsp vanilla
1/2 tsp coconut extract
¼ cup chopped nuts (walnuts or pecans)
1/3 cup cranberries
1/3 cup raisins
¼ cup shredded coconut
¼ cup water (if needed)
¼ tsp cinnamon (helps lower blood pressure)

Instructions

Place almond flour, coconut flour flax salt and baking soda in a food processor
Pulse ingredients together
Pulse in eggs, oil honey and vinegar
Transfer batter to a greased 7.5 x 3.5 loaf pan
Bake at 350 for 30 minutes, take out of pan and cool on a rack
Can be frozen as a full loaf or in slices.

I really missed cereal for breakfast, I love cereal, but it doesn't always agree with me. I found myself hungry in the middle of the morning. Whenever I eat protein for breakfast, I wasn't hungry. I didn't want to eat bacon and eggs every morning, but I wanted the protein. I found this recipe for Paleo Bread that contains protein in the eggs, the quinoa flour, and the nuts. I found it fully satisfies me for the entire morning. A friend of mine at this bread before she worked out, and found it gave her energy.

I put this bread in a container in the fridge, and cut of a ½ in slice every morning. I have done this for months, and it is delicious and I never get tired of it.

Chocolate Chia Seed Pudding

Serves 2

1-¼ Cup coconut milk

¼ Cup chia seeds

3 tbs. cocoa powder

¼ tsp. Himalayan Sea Salt

1 tbs. maple syrup

Optional add ins/toppings: crystallized ginger, goji berries, nut butter, coconut, fresh citrus, bananas, nuts, pomegranate seeds, whipped coconut cream.

Instructions

Add all the ingredients to a glass jar with a lid. Give it a quick stir and then cover with the lid, shake until all ingredients are well combined. Refrigerate for at least 4 hours or overnight, until very thick and pudding like. Serve chilled with whatever toppings you like.

Part Seven:

Factors Influencing Your Journey

"I love the power of being in charge"

Emotional Integrity
Once you know, you can't pretend you don't know.

- Drinking many cups of coffee per day with cream and sugar adds about 1000 calories to your daily intake. It makes your body very acidic, which allows cancer cells to flourish in some cases. Your body needs an Acid/Alkaline balance to be healthy. If you drink too much coffee and your system is very acidic, and it may inhibit your efforts to release weight.

- Eating most Granola bars is similar to eating a chocolate bar. You are NOT eating something healthy. You need to read the label and find out exactly what you are eating. Items that are healthy typically have five ingredients or less and you are able to pronounce them all.

- Buy unsweetened Yogurt and sweeten it yourself. If it is already sweetened, it likely has ingredients you don't want or that are not good for you – like fructose. If you sweeten Yogurt with pure Maple Syrup, or raw unpasteurized honey, or ground up dates or prunes, it will be very sweet and good for you. The less foreign ingredients we put into our body the better.

- Just because it says "Gluten Free" does not mean it is healthy. The food industry uses the term as a marketing tool. I have found the label Gluten Free on : potato chips, bacon, corn on the cob, meat in a package. These items don't have gluten in them to begin with. The food industry counts on you picking it up thinking you are helping yourself to a product that will benefit you.

- Bagels are not a healthy breakfast choice. **They are dough.** Adding some cream cheese does NOT add enough protein to make them a beneficial choice. It could be the reason you get hungry just a few hours later.

- Lobster, Shrimp and fried Calamari, is not what is meant by adding seafood to your diet.

- All fruit smoothies spike your blood sugar and too much natural sugar adds calories and can make your system acidic. When your system is too acidic, you crave carbohydrates in baked goods etc.

- Double double in coffee or tea isn't beneficial for your body or your health. Examine why you need so much in order to have a coffee or tea. Do you not like the flavour of coffee and are trying to mask it? Thousands of unwanted and unneeded calories consumed – why? Gradually lessen each on and see how the flavour bursts and you might find you quite like it.

Elsa Notarandrea
RHN Nutritional Consultant
Brantford, ON

Visit the website for recipes, information and health.
www.beautyoffood.ca
elsa@beautyoffood.ca
519.732.5820

In the 25 years that I have known Jo-Anne, I have only seen love and compassion given to everyone around her. I have seen her grow spiritually and she has such a gift of sharing.

Jo-Anne's main focus, apart from being a wonderful wife, mother, grandmother and friend to people, is teaching people how to love and forgive oneself and those around them. When I started "Beauty of Food" she showed me how to have faith in myself and helped me see that I was on the right path and "that I could do it"! Because I trusted her, I knew that my love of cooking and nutritional knowledge, I could be an extension of the psychological aspect of this program.

VGB and Exhale Weight's "gift" is to eat less. Three meals a day, stop when you are full and no snacking in between.
So you are eating less!!!   *WHAT ARE YOU EATING?*

As a nutritionist my main goal is to empower the individual in their kitchen. Cooking quick easy meals packed with dense nutrition eliminates any feeling of deprivation.

I try and take into consideration, that everyone is unique with different likes and dislikes, lifestyles and health concerns. While I help you *incorporate* fresh, local, organic ingredients, my **main** goal is to get you cooking.

I like to start *you* with a few healthy staples such as good quality salt and sugar, oil, organic eggs etc… You can all do this, some at faster pace than others…. but it is at your pace. I certainly did it an ingredient at a time. I will start *you* at the point you are at, with what you are cooking right now

- Never cook
- Rarely cook
- Cook but not a lot
- Enhance what you already know how to cook but even healthier

This becomes your personal best. In my cooking class I will show you quick simple meals. Each person will participate and best of all, you get to eat at my dining room table and take the leftovers home!!

Jo-Anne and I might have different viewpoints on some aspects, but the bottom line the two of us are focusing on the Body, Mind and Spirit…it all works together.

If one aspect is off, it seems that the rest becomes off balance. Once the individual finds out what the root of the problem is, then they can concentrate on the food habits which has been the "comfort food", feeding the negative emotions…. leading you to this program.

About Beauty of Food ~ Elsa Notarandrea

My name is Elsa Notarandrea a Registered Holistic Nutritionist; I graduated from Canadian School of Natural Nutrition, where I was nominated Valedictorian of my class.

I am a wife to a wonderful husband Ezio of over 32 years, a mother of two beautiful adult children and spouses and a best friend to my dog Lolla.

I grew up with first generation Italian immigrants where food was, and still is, the core of the family. As a child I did not feel well after our meals, I know now that gluten played a big role in this. I was never sick enough for a doctor, but it gave me a very sluggish feel and made it very hard to concentrate. Even though homemade *Pasta and Bread* was served at almost all of our four course meals, we also had good quality, nutritious foods along with it. We had a garden full of greens and other vegetables every year. Being that my grandparents lived with us, my mother and grandmother did all the cooking. I never cooked a day in my life.

Imagine me in my young adult married life (married at 19 years old), never having cooked, all I could handle was cooking one-course meals, because cooking like my mother and grandmother, I felt was too complicated. My meals consisted of mainly refined empty calorie meals (mainly gluten filled), toast, local donuts (oh they were so good), pizza, sandwiches, and lets not forget the *Pasta* (a Celiacs' nightmare). So if I thought I did not feel well when I lived with my parents, it only got worse when I was cooking myself. I came up with a simple solution.... skip breakfast and lunch and eat around 2pm, at least I could get my work done. So as the months and years went by my bad eating habits was taxing my body. I had never told my family I didn't feel well because for me it was normal.

We had our son when I was 20 and our daughter when I was 22, and then at 23, my husband and I started a new business. Through those years with a young family and busy lifestyle, the iron in my body was very low and my husband got gout (hereditary). Being the main cook, it became quite a challenge for me to cook for us. Where I needed foods that provided iron, a lot of those foods were high in purines (what my husband had to avoid), and also pleasing the children. I was

36 when my mother at the age of 60 died of stomach cancer (her mother and brother also died of stomach cancer), I started to think, there HAS to be a connection with food.

So my journey began, with my Italian background and love of food, I knew I could tweak our family recipes and make them more nutritious, while maintaining my Mom and Nonna's authenticity. I found that the foods beauty could be nourishing and healing just by using wholesome ingredients. I am now able to rotate and balance meat, grains and a rainbow of vegetables at every meal, keeping the meals quick and simple.

Quality is key!! With **your** determination, I can help **you** improve your quality of life through good **nutritious meals**, with the support of some supplements, along with a good exercise program (walking, weights, yoga, meditation…). Vitamin **F** is the best vitamin there is, ingredients: Good quality *F*ood, **F**amily and **F**riends. Getting back to the table with family and friends is not only good for the soul but for the body, mind and spirit.

The **Heart of Good Nutrition** is the **Beauty of Food**.

Beauty of Food offers:

Group Nutritional Hands-on Cooking Class (4 - 6 people) 2-3 hour Cooking Session
- Casual gathering of 4 - 6 people (family, friends, co-workers etc.)
- Location provided by Beauty of Food
- Class includes most foods (minimal charge for certain meat products)

☐ *Menu could reflect a topic such as:*
      o Improving **digestion**

- o **Detox** (preparing meals for your detox)
- o Controlling **blood sugar** (foods best to help stabilize)
- o **Inflammation** friendly foods
- o **Gluten free** balanced meals
- o **Grains** (incorporating alternative grains)
- o **Protein** (not just meat)

☐ *Best nutrients from each meal:*
- o Breakfast
- o Lunch
- o Dinner
- o Appetizers/Snacks
- o Bulk prepared foods (weekly menus)

☐ *Seasonal Cooking getting the best nutrients from each season:*
- o Winter (warming foods)
- o Spring (cleansing food)
- o Summer (cooling foods)
- o Fall (harvesting foods)
- o Year-round meals (such as apples, sweet potato, rutabaga, sprouts, onions, mushrooms, carrots, cabbage)

One-on-One Nutrition and Wellness Consultation

1st Session/Class (3 hours): We will discuss aspects of your current diet such as sensitivities, selection, etc...
- Includes cooking session.

Follow-up Session or Sessions (2 hours/session): Cooking class/es with nutritional facts covering one or a combination of breakfast, lunch, supper and snack

Elsa Notarandrea RHN, Nutritional Consultant
Brantford, ON
www.beautyoffreed.ca
elsa@beautyoffood.ca

Phone 519 732 5820

Relationships

Our entire life is filled with Relationships. We have a relationship with our parents, siblings, grandparents, cousins, spouses, children, grandchildren, pets and ourselves.

Friends, our boss, co-workers, customers, and others we do day to day business with are also relationships and all the relationships.

If you play a sport, you have a relationship with the coach or if you are coach, you have a relationship with your team.

There are a lot of factors that can cause parts of those relationships to be other than the way we wish, hope, or want them to be, including ourselves.

The most important relationship we have is with our own self. Your body image, criticizing yourself, calling yourself names, berating yourself, lecturing yourself, are behaviours that we probably do not do to others. Somehow, we think we are improving our self if we blame or shame ourselves. Perhaps we are just carrying on where some other significant relationship left off.

Stress is the result of insisting things be other than the way they are.

What is the best way to juggle and handle all these relationships? We often fall into the trap of wanting to please everyone else and forget ourselves. Relationships begin with you. If you love yourself, like yourself, and can be fully be happy with no one else but you, it is likely that outside relationships are happy and healthy as well.

The most prominent relationship for most people is with a spouse. Think back to when you are dating. Remember all the preparation to smell good, to look good, to act well that we did to impress and to want to make them like us.

Once we have been in a relationship for a period of time, we are comfortable enough that our spouse can see us at our worst and will still love us. Isn't that what our vows say – for better or worse? Is that what it means? I don't thinks so.

When we are dating we are able to filter our mouth. When we have been married for a while, we think we can say and do hurtful things and it won't matter. If you wouldn't say the words to your best friend, then don't say it. I can remember once when my husband said something to me – so insignificant that I can't even remember what it was but it stung at the time. I asked him "Would you have said that to –John your best friend?

My goal is not to point out my husbands faults. It is just where I am drawing my experiences.

An old woman was sipping on a glass of wine while sitting on the patio with her husband of 50+ years. She says "I love you so much, I don't know how I could ever live without you"
Her husband asks "Is that you or the wine talking?"
She answered, " That's me talking to the wine"

Another time, during an argument, my husband said "Well that's just stupid" He didn't call me stupid, but that is the way I heard and perceived it. My answer to him was "If I am the stupidest person on the face of the earth, then I have a right to be the stupidest person on the face of the earth and you don't have the right to tell me I can't. " He opened his mouth to say something back, but then just shook his head and said he couldn't argue with that. That is as close as I get to "I was wrong"

Saying "I was wrong, I'm sorry" for some people are words that don't flow easily. Start saying it, practice it and it will get easier. We would say it to our best friend.

Treat your family like company and your company like family. Think about that for a moment. When company comes, we are on our best behaviour, and we filter our words. If we do that with family, life gets easier.

We often snap at our children when we are rushed or overwhelmed with tasks. I think every Mother has had those days when we go into our children's bedroom at night when they are sleeping and wonder why we were so short with them that day. Forgive yourself and move on.

Accepting

Many times we just wish to win the argument and be right. I am a right fighter from way back. I had to learn to let go. Let go. Let go. I still fall into the trap at times. Old patterns and behaviours emerge just when you think you have got it conquered.

It is a constant practice in pulling back and saying to yourself "Oh well" The reward is you just feel better.

Most anything in life feels better by letting go. Many people in the world today subconsciously feel hopeless and helpless at the unfairness of the world. It is not something we consciously feel. We lament and talk about it and it causes stress.

- Big government that seems to make their own rules.
- Big business that seems to forget the average everyday person.
- Crime is taking over.
- Everyway we turn, there is a tax.
- Negative news
- Added made up charges on just about every bill

Gosh, I am feeling pressure just writing this. A lovely wise friend pointed out to me to let go and make peace with the way the world is, stop pushing up the hill.

Multi-tasking has become a way of life. Relationships can often get caught in the middle of us just getting so busy, many couples make the time for each other the way they did when they first met. Date night once a week is crucial to a happy relationship. Nothing should interfere, no matter how important we think it is, with keeping the date each week at the same time.

We need new ways to manage our lives without the typical fight, flight or freeze responses, which drain our ability to function at 100%.

Fight, flight or freeze was a way for ancient peoples to cope with lurking danger that appeared out of nowhere. You could fight the dinosaur, freeze and hope you were invisible or run for your life. The Adrenal gland gave you a squirt of adrenalin to accomplish whichever one you chose.

In today's world where that danger isn't present and daily stress has become "normal", our Adrenals are just constantly leaking small amounts of adrenalin trying to help us cope. Adrenal fatigue is a common ailment many don't even know they have.

Everyone has issues in their life; so what are we going to do about them? When someone has a festering sore, and instead of going to the doctor, or finding an ointment or finding a solution, they let it get worse. When you have an emotional issue, and you leave it festering, the result is the same; it gets worse. Could Relaxation Hypnosis be the answer?

Take a moment and put the palm of your hand on the end of your nose with your fingers spread. That is how you see your own stuff. Now, move your hand away from your face and look at how you can see the details of your hand more clearly.

By choosing a Hypnotist, the very act of relaxation begins the process of lightening your load and moving the mountain. The Hypnotist helps you step back from the drama and chaos, and see it clearly from a different perspective and viewpoint.

When you're buried in your problems, the pile feels futile and never ending. When you avoid one issue, another issue crops up and adds to the pile. You then step into a role of the mouse, looking at everything from a tiny perspective, instead of flying high above it all and looking down to see where help and solutions could be. Being in Hypnosis, the very benefit of relaxation helps you to see the pile from the Hawks perspective.

Being in Hypnosis feels like the feeling you have just moments before you drop off to sleep. You may realize that you forgot to get the clothes out of the dryer (or something equally unimportant), but you are so relaxed, you just don't care; so you let it go and sink into the feeling. Everyone describes it differently, but the relaxation is the same for everyone.

Relaxation can be felt as a heaviness of the limbs, a tingling sensation in your hands or feet, or it can feel like you are floating. Most people experience heaviness - loose, limp and relaxed but all agree that it is a delicious feeling to have complete relaxation. It allows us to realize just how tense we are daily as we go about the tasks of the day.

When you come out of Hypnosis, that feeling of relaxation and calmness stays with you so that the beginning of resolving problems small or large doesn't seem like such a daunting task. We start with relaxation to begin a new path and a new way of looking at things.

Imagine date night after you and your significant other have both had a general relaxation Hypnosis session and then proceed to have dinner and a movie - or perhaps just skip the movie?

A stepparent doesn't just marry a spouse: they marry their spouse's entire situation.
They have to find a balance between supporting and defending without overstepping invisible and visible boundaries

Top Five Ways to Raise Your Mood and Get Out of the Muck.

Muck is a light hearted term to describe when we are feeling blue or grumpy. In this hurry up, keep up world, fast food, drive through "everything", too many of our days are punctuated with intense longing, a missing sense of magic and unconditional joy. This longing manifests itself into strong moments of unwanted stress, sadness, anger, frustration and fear. What we focus on expands and the more we wallow in the muck, the more muck we have, and the more we create.

Would it surprise you to know that the planetary shifts that are taking place can make you feel as if you are scattered and disconnected? If the planetary shifts can create the turbulent weather all over the world, it makes sense that our energy bodies can be affected as well.

Suggestions for shifting your thinking, your mood and your vibration

1. *Acknowledge the emotion* Say to yourself "Hello anger, old friend. Thank you for showing up right now. I am grateful that I can express myself and not stuff it down because when I do that, it makes me feel like my opinion doesn't matter and therefore, I don't matter."

Now use that wonderful imagination to see the anger leaving your body and your mind in any way that pops into your thoughts. Perhaps it escapes like a puff of smoke. Perhaps it leaves with the exhale of a deep breath. Get creative and see it leaving disguised in a costume or a like a cartoon character stomping off because you won't let it stay. This allows the emotion to be freely expressed and released, creating a space for you to move into JOY. Sounds silly to be imagining this doesn't it? That is the whole point. Getting silly lightens your mood instantly and brings a smile.

2. *Allow yourself up to 2 minutes* (set a timer) to stay in the muck just feeling how yucky it is. Your thoughts are very powerful so imagine yourself in a mud pit moving and pushing and pulling to extract yourself out of the stuck feeling. Never before has it been so important to flow with your emotions by surrendering to the feeling. Once you truly feel the muck, it becomes easier to then imagine freeing yourself easily and effortlessly.

3. ***Discover the feeling of freedom*** Conquering the task and leaving the muck, and choose JOY. Choose it by imagining it is an item in a store and you are putting it into your cart. Put JOY on as if it is an item of clothing or a lotion that could be spread on yourself. Imagine it is a cloak and wrap around your shoulders leaving you feeling warm, protected and light.

4. ***Get the energy flowing in your body***; Walk, sing, dance, stretch, or exercise,. Look in a mirror. Look deeply into your eyes and tell yourself "I love you". Smile and allow that smile to become a chuckle still looking into your eyes.

5. ***Play with a pet***, or groom and pet them and feel the connection. Animals are evolving as rapidly as we are and often sense our needs and can lift and change our moods.

With this new awareness, be open to what's going on energetically in the weather and on the planet and know that it affects your energy body and how you can remain balanced through the turmoil.

Quieting your mind and using your imagination is the basis of self-hypnosis. We daydream, or find our mind wandering daily. Regular practice of meditation or self-hypnosis using these simple, fun techniques allows you to spend more time in JOY than in muck.

Part Eight:

Testimonials

"This is the easiest thing I've ever done"
This is the statement I hear the most from clients

A Colleagues Weight Journey with VGB

Everyone can get testimonials and if we think about it, the testimonial is only important to the person who experiences it and the person like myself, who receives it. They are interesting but if you are not getting those results yourself, a testimonial can make you feel "Why aren't I feeling like that? Why isn't that happening to me? "

I once attended a course on enhancing your website and the teacher recommended putting testimonials on the website so people would know you are successful. She suggested that at first you just make them up yourself – who would know? **I would know!**

I asked Les, a Hypnosis graduate of mine if he wanted to attend the Sheila Granger Virtual Gastric Band with Hypnosis course with me. The first thing we did at the course was stand up and introduce ourselves. When it was time for Les to speak, he said, " I was a fat baby, a fat little boy, a fat teenager and now I am a fat man. I have never known in my entire life what so called NORMAL weight is." "I am looking forward to learning this and helping myself and others with their weight" His brutal honesty in front of this entire class shocked me and I knew he had come to a crossroads in his life.

When we returned home, we practiced the technique – installing the Virtual Gastric band on each other and then began to see clients. Each one of us were immediately impressed with how we felt and how our clients were responding.

Les has type 2 diabetes but does not want to go on the medication or follow the diet recommended by his physician. Always a rebel. Even though I have put his experience in the book, I am not recommending that anyone not follow a doctors advice or do what Les did because they read it here. He takes his own blood sugar

reading several times throughout the day. He explained to me that the safe zone reading is between 5 – 7. This is a Canadian number, I believe in the US and perhaps other places in the world it might be different. When we began Les was getting readings throughout the day around 15 + and at times spiking into the 20's – very dangerous.

Below are observations from Les

September 14, 2012   First time in about two years my blood sugar went to 9.0 fasting this morning.   And I still do not take the pills I am supposed to or do the dietary hospital diet advice thing.

I was creeping up to 15 to 18 on the blood meter, which is very bad with spikes into the 20's
It is 5 to 7 that is called normal

So I dropped an average of 5 to 8 points already in 5 months with VGB/Exhale Weight lifestyle
So norm level for me by Halloween is do-able **I feel the no snacking between meals is the ticket to success.** And that is my story.

Les

January 2013

I gave up on most grains in May   [really hard at the time.]
A lot of stuff cleared up within days. Then it was easy to stop grains.
I get into breaded stuff with wheat or gravies with flour as thickener.
Once in a while ….I feel it
New Year's Day had two big Macs only first time in a year because McDonalds was the only place open after we finished our fireworks show. This is routine after a 16-hour physical day when we work right

through mealtimes - you are so hungry you do not care. Tired and sleepy

This time I still am bloated up big time still feel uncomfortable after 5 days.
Yes - you keep getting more sensitive as you go.
It is not the gluten only part. There are other irritants in grains that bother people too.
Plus GMO junk in there and a part that never gets talked about is the molds and fungus that lives on the outside of the wheat grain.   I suggest you get into once in a while to keep your body defenses up and running. Rice and corn once in a while too.

Gluten free cookies fire me up the same as the real thing – I am sensitive them also.

Les

May 2013

You know a year ago my blood sugars were up to 18+. Not good.
Now a year latter no pills, no needles , no doctor interferences
Blood sugar is 7.7 this morning. (Target 5 to 7)
Any time you are over 10 the kidneys' get damaged and leak out minerals.
When you get 20 + your body and brain life is reduced and chance of death really good.

My buddies laugh at me and I feel sorry for them. They followed doctor's orders to the tee yet are getting worse.
They all go on about eating more often. Little snacks many meals, with pills and needles at each meal. Their sugars are at 15+. Health falling apart.

Too bad they mentally do not stop and take a personal assessment of themselves. Like a quality control check in a factory.

If you do this, what happens? If you do that, what happens?

If the small snacks between meals is keeping sugar levels up. Try something different for a while.

Each and every one that I seen have not let their blood sugars levels drop low enough to start to use up body fat up.

Les

September 2013

First time in about two years my blood sugar went to 9.0 fasting this morning. And I still do not take the pills I am suppose to. And do the dietary hospital diet advice thing. I was creeping up to 15 to 18 on the blood meter, which is very bad with spikes into the +20s. It is 5 to 7 is called normal

So I dropped an average of 5 to 8 points already in 5 months with VGB lifestyle. So norm level for me is by Halloween is do-able

I feel the no snacking between meals in the ticket to success.

Les

Conclusion

Les was the one who figured out for the Exhale Weight Program, which uses Sheila Grangers protocol of three small meals a day – just those three small meals a day why it works. It is the way we used to eat in the 50's and 60's when there was little fast food and meals were ate at home. The average adult in the family had a diet that was about 1500 calories a day. Incredible but true.

Les was the one that looked up the information to add to what he already knew. When digestion finishes from breakfast, which takes about three hours, the liver begins on the fat stores. When digestion finishes from lunch, the liver begins on the fat stores. When digestion finishes from dinner, the liver can work on the fat stores all night long while you sleep. Anytime to eat something in between meals or snack and graze at night, the body has to process and digest it instead of working on the fat stores. Intermittent fasting.

The Exhale Weight Program, which is partnered with Sheila Grangers Virtual Gastric Band with Hypnosis, is not a quick weight loss result. Time goes by so quickly these days. Would it be ok if in a year you got the results you wanted? Or in a year you just realized that this is an easy and healthy lifestyle for life because you feel better?

This program does not weigh or measure the clients. I think it is humiliating. It can also be discouraging when you think you have had a really good week and the scale doesn't support it. I would rather someone FEEL their pants getting looser or be able to get into one size smaller OR as Les does it – he hikes his belt in another notch. He is still wearing the same belt from when he started and has hiked it in 5 belt loops and has the worn notches to prove it.

I tell him all the time that he is a walking testimonial.

Jo-Anne

Support emails to my clients

First Session Review
At the first session, we went over two concepts – Who is in charge?
Who is in control?
Did you hang up your "I am in Control sign"

Body Image Exercise – You probably have done the body image
exercise by now. Be aware of what comes up in your thinking.

Did you listen to your cd cither in the morning or at night? It is
important to reinforce Hypnosis.

In the middle of the morning or afternoon, when your habit of getting
hungry comes up – did you go and brush your teeth and drink water?
What happened?

Jo-Anne

I took a hypnosis course on **stress** yesterday that was one of the most
informative, interesting, informational and helpful course and will fit
right in with Exhale Weight and clients who want to quit smoking.

Many in the Exhale Weight program say they eat because of stress,
they eat something to relax.

I have a client coming this week who said she quit smoking herself
and then went back to it after three years. When I asked her why she
went back after such a long time, she answered – stress. I smoke to
relax when I'm stressed.

Since nicotine and sugar are stimulants, it is hard to see how putting stimulants in the body will relax someone physically, so we hear that phrase "comfort food"

Food is not the enemy; we need to eat to nourish the body, not to soothe the soul.

Thank-you all for the interesting emails telling me about your insights doing the body image exercise and other thoughts and feeling that have come up in this first week. One person wrote they went farther than the mirror exercise and did the "I love you" "I love you" "I love you" "I love you" "I love you" patting her body all over and then looked deep into her own eyes and said "I LOVE YOU"

She said, **"It felt wonderful"**

This program is to get you back to where you love and accept yourself now. It is a major key to the success.

Jo-Anne

One question that has come up is that one participant found her mind wandering during the hypnosis session. Everyone experiences the Hypnosis in a different way but I actually want your conscious mind to wander or rest or not care what is going on. She has a lot of red in her home and knew something was supposed to happen when she saw red but couldn't remember what. This is great as your subconscious mind does remember and will carry out what you need to do as automatically as blinking or a heartbeat.

When you are driving, every once in awhile you see a cute personalized licence plate or bumper sticker. Your **conscious mind** In order to notice this particular licence plate, (because it is different and stands out) means your **subconscious mind** has also recorded every other licence plate. Isn't that interesting?

If you go to a coffee shop every morning five days a week, and just buy a coffee – nothing else – totalling $1.70, the total for a year is $442.00. If you are periodically purchasing a donut, bagel, breakfast sandwich or cookie, that amount doubles or triples. If you are periodically buying lunch that total becomes much higher – between $2,000 and $ 3,000. Add up what you spend per day, x 7 days, x 4 weeks x 12 months. What else could you do with that money? Yesterday morning, one participant had written a fairly long email with some really good observations and questions. I answered her personally and then went to have a shower. I get most of my ideas in the shower for some reason and it popped into my mind that I had not noticed something in her email. Here is an excerpt that has a message that I missed at first.

I haven't and don't usually suffer with hunger pangs mid morning or afternoon so it hasn't been an issue for me in the past. However, **I've learned to be a grazer** with fruit, veggies, or yogurt. Yesterday, I felt **starved** about an hour before lunchtime yesterday but was on the road running an errand. I don't ever stop in for a treat or drink so this wasn't an issue for me. I waited until I got home for a healthy meal.

Two things come to mind in that paragraph. I asked her to be mindful of her words as she "felt starved". I suggested that she use a different word to acknowledge it. You could say, I feel like I want a little something. Starving brings to mind that we must eat a lot to stave off or satisfy with a large amount of food and wolf it down. She does mention that she doesn't stop as a rule but sometimes this program will wake the beast within and you will find yourself thinking about it more because we ARE being more aware of what we are doing. In North America, people are not starving.

The second and most important "aha" in that paragraph is that I noticed that she "waited until she got home" I immediately emailed her back to say that I hoped she felt very powerful as "SHE WAS IN CONTROL" not the food. That is why it is SO important to make copies of " I am in Control" and hang them around the house. She had indicated to me she had done that and there was one copy hanging in almost every room of her house.

This was my answer to her after my shower -
I just had a shower and is occurred to me that when you waited until you came home to satisfy that starving feeling, this is the first experience of "I am in control of what I eat, **when I eat**, and how much I eat. **I would like you to sit and close your eyes and think that through and check in with how powerful and in control that feels and how much you LIKE that feeling.**

Weight and why we overeat is a complicated issue and it is difficult for me to try to get all the concepts to you in one session. You can see from the few brief emails that already there are reactions and observations and questions.

Jo-Anne

For some people, reading the emails I'm sending out is helpful. It comes in small doses instead of trying to understand it all in one sitting.

For those who have decided to NOT continue on the program, you have a choice to receive the emails or not. If you don't wish to receive them, and have decided not to continue on the remainder of the program, just reply to this email with "please take me off the list"

I don't get offended and I don't take it personally, so please don't feel that you will hurt my feelings or I will be angry or offended.

If you have decided **not** to continue on the program and try it on your own, but WANT to read the emails, that is ok with me. I think other people's experiences are valuable to everyone in their weight journey. You are already on the list and I just click to send out the email. There is no extra work involved for me.

Jo-Anne

One of the questions coming up is about the Hypnosis. I explained that your mind wandering is actually a good thing because while the conscious mind is not judging and analyzing, the subconscious mind will absorb everything.

The question coming up is "I think I fell asleep – you were talking and then I couldn't hear you" "I even at one point thought I was snoring."

The way you know if you were sleeping or not is: if you come up and open your eyes on the count when everyone else does. The light snoring is because your throat and pallet become so relaxed. Others will wipe their eyes as they come out of hypnosis because the eyes are very relaxed and the tear ducts will flow.

One family is having so much fun with asking each other "Who is in charge?" and then laughing. I hope all of you will approach this program light-heartedly.

Jo-Anne

Our family is having fun with it asking each other "Who is in charge?" and then laughing. I hope all of you will approach this program light-heartedly.

Jo-Anne

It has been a very busy week and weekend. Do you ever notice that when you are very busy you are preoccupied with what you are doing and food hardly ever enters your mind? We often work right through a meal and are surprised when we feel hungry and look at the clock and say to ourselves "No wonder, lunch was an hour ago"

On Saturday, I travelled to Bellville (three hour drive) to the Canadian Society of Dowsers convention. I got up at 5:00 am and had breakfast at 6:00 am while I drove down that morning. I was sitting in the lecture hall and about 11:00 am, and feeling hungry. There was no food anywhere and lunch was served at 12 Noon. I knew there was no food anywhere for another hour and so the thought was easily dismissed. You have all experienced this and yet when food is available it is just as easy to justify eating and not waiting one more hour. **I actually felt very pleased with myself** as I sipped some water and tuned back in to what the speaker was saying.

I have received a few emails about making better choices and how much that makes you feel in control. Feeling in control is heady and powerful and just feels good. I like that feeling. Are you surprised how good that feels and how much you like it?

One lady who leads a very busy lifestyle (don't we all) works out of town full time, has a family, and regularly eats fast food. She emailed me the following:

*I had a great week even with being busy at work. I was late getting into town so I stopped by Wendy's on the way home to grab a quick dinner. Normally I would of gone overboard with a large burger fries, drink, and a frosty. This week when I stopped at Wendy's, **I surprised myself,** by changing my order to a small chili and a small salad instead which I was still not able to finish fully when I did sit down to eat.*

Reading her email, I can hear and feel her pride and power of being in control after the initial surprise of ordering less and still not finishing everything.

GOOD JOB - I AM PROUD OF YOU

We can immediately jump to judgment and say "Fast food is empty calories and has a lot of salt, sugar and chemicals" **It doesn't matter.** This program, Exhale Weight - you eat what you want, as long as it is three small meals a day. The phenomena that happens **later** is that you start to make even better choices as you continue. This was the first step. Baby steps to get to where you want. The entire key is feeling IN CONTROL and not deprived of ANYTHING as long as it is within those three small meals a day.

This was a major leap forward for this lady.

You have probably noticed by now that I repeat "three small meals a day" **I have received emails that tell me you don't think of food constantly the way you used to.** The subconscious mind will let go and dismiss thoughts that are not relevant to the moment. The subconscious mind records them and can recall them , but for the moment can let them go. The conscious mind also dismisses thoughts that are not needed because we have so many. **Because you have established and cemented three small meals a day,** the subconscious mind says " I just had breakfast, the next thing is lunch, that is completed, so I don't have to think about that right now"

That is not exactly how it works – it is not the scientific way it works, but I always try to put ideas into a form that you can instantly understand without thinking about it.

Who has time to figure out the subconscious mind?
Don't worry – be happy

Jo-Anne

So that is an example of the support emails that I use with the Exhale Weight program.

Emails From My Clients

Jo-Anne! Wow! We can't believe how amazing all of this is with the hypnosis and the food with Elsa! Our eating habits have changed significantly, our cravings diminished, and our bodies are shifting into healthier, more comfortable shapes.

You have done wonders for us in such a short period of time. We feel better and happier! Our life does not revolve around food as a distraction now, and, a distraction it was! Being free from cravings and habits that have been laid to rest, well, it's a miracle! How could that happen to simply and quickly! Who would have known! Not me! Not this easy. Not even so much the feeling of fullness (which we do feel!), but the biggest thing is not missing any of those foods that we craved and that railroaded us everyday! We DO crave veggies and healthy foods now, naturally! Isn't that WILD!!!

We had the pure joy and pleasure of attending Elsa's food class last night. Shouldn't be called "nutritious", should JUST be called "delicious"!!! Wow, I've always wanted to know how to cook incredible RAW meals without it taking "raw", and man oh man, did she EVER show us mouth watering, eye celebrating, soul soothing dishes! Who ever knew!!! Chocolate pudding to boot! Can you believe it…made with raw avocado! Isn't that out of this world! We LOVE that girl, and I am addicted to attending more of her classes to learn how to have that "PARTY IN YOUR MOUTH" as you call it, and party it is! (to be honest, I thought you were exaggerating a wee bit, but, heavens no! You called that one!) We did wraps with rice paper with veggie and the most succulent chicken my mouth has ever experienced! We made so many different exciting things last night! I could go on and on! This was an education that I really needed to know, but simply didn't know where to get this information around here! Elsa makes everything so easy and DO-ABLE!

She has gotten both Rick and I excited about the prospects of Raw food, and how easily It can be incorporated into our lives, without being salad after salad! We loved Elsa and her passion for healthy food. The girl is simply a food-genius!

Jo-Anne, Rick and I want to thank you so much for enhancing our lives and saving our health. You are a magical wizard", and I say that with the most love and respect I could ever say to any one! Thank you!!!

Cherie and Rick

Good Morning Jo-Anne!

You probably get these daily messages, but this one reminds me of you, and something that you would say. It also triggers why some of us do better with this new gastro band that perhaps others. I just had to share this with you this morning. I love resonating with your vibration. I always feel so happy and content and energetic around your energy!!! From the bottom of my heart, with deep gratitude, thank you!!! Another successful day ahead of us, and I'm so excited.
AND A BIG PS WOMAN TO WOMAN....
Not sure what you did, but my husband FINALLY has got his "sexy back"!!! Thus, no more night snacking...hmm, go figure! I LOVE YOU!!! (and we're talking well over a decade!!!!) Don't know what you did, but keep on doing it!!! Big smiles at my house!

What the heck did you do to me?....Ha-ha!...LOL

I'm the English girl that came to Brantford from London last week for the virtual gastric by pass. I bought your book and you were kind enough to sign it for me. I was fascinated by your colleague Elsa and would love to do some work with her too.

I absolutely LOVE the book. Have been reading and using a few techniques. Love your voice on the CD, you sent me off into LA LA Land again last night. I woke up about 2 in the morning with an ear bud stuck to my face. Painful. Ha-ha!

I have heard about this program on Dr. Oz. There is an English hypnotist, Paul McLean, I think his name is, who uses hypnotherapy for all sorts of wonderful things. I have his book on weight loss but never got around to reading and getting serious about it. He was on again about 3 moths ago and he was talking about virtual gastric bypass surgery. My ears pricked up then he said he was working in the states and it was not available just yet…but soon. Then you emailed me.
Coincidence…I think not….

Well I love this program…can't believe how full I am. I seem to be able to eat only small meals and if I go over…don't feel good. I absolutely believe this program is going to help a lot of people.
I would love to continue this program but I don't have $400 up front. I can do this in two payments thought $200 now and a post dated cheque for $200 on October 15th. Would you consider this?
Not sure if anyone else from London is going to sign up. Please let me know. And thank you, thank you, and thank you for bringing this to me.

I would not mind repeating session 1. Any reinforcement is great. Offer open for session 1 as well.

Tuesday I picked at my food. I had my usual oatmeal for breakfast with a cup of tea. About 10:00 am. I was a little peckish and I ate a tofu mango dessert (like a yogurt) The last few spoonful's I was struggling with…then around noon I ate once slice of bread and a cup of tea…not hungry…I barely ate anything for supper. The following days same thing…till Friday around 5:00pm. I had a craving for a pork chop so we went out to dinner and I ate the chop, the veggies and the baked potato. The most I had eaten at one meal all week. Saturday I picked in the day and was out to dinner again with girlfriends. We went to Swiss Chalet. I was worried about what to eat so instead of the ¼ chicken dinner I had a salad with a chicken breast. It had walnuts, feta cheese, raisins, mandarins, lettuce, it was huge. I brought half home in a doggy bag. At the restaurant I noticed I ate two of the little rolls with butter and loved the taste of the butter. When I got home about an hour and a half later I ate another roll with butter and savoured the butter… I don't know why… maybe it was the salt or something…I don't use salt normally.

I just checked on the scale and I think I may have lost a pound of two…probably because I went out to eat twice this weekend. I do think I need reinforcement right now.
I feel I am slipping…I definitely think I overrode my stomach on Friday.

Anyway today I have had 2 cups of tea so far…I don't drink much water…and a bowl of oatmeal and I am full.
Looking forward to seeing you soon.

Patti

Hi Jo-Anne

Just an update

Thank you so much for your help
I have had a great week so far; I never thought I'd be free from
thinking of nothing but food that rules my life.

I have not had a drink of Pepsi since Tuesday

I think it was so funny I didn't feel like water before I left the session
but I can tell you by the time I got home, I had a bottle of water in
front of me. I did fell like drinking pop, so I just went with it.

I haven't had a lot of bottles per day, but I have had the water bottle so
much beside me, I've been carrying it around with me everywhere.

I listen to the cd's daily faithfully

It was funny when I got in the car from our session I put the cd in the
cd player on my way home so I could listen to the daily one while
driving, well it took the cd and wouldn't play, I had to get my husband
to get it out. So needless to say my cd player in the car does not work .
I will know that for the next time. □
I just listen to them at home.

Sometimes I am a little hungry before I go to bed, but I don't feel the
need to eat.

I am down 2 lbs. and a bit, I am sure if I stay true to our sessions I will
loose more

I have a long road to go, when I have to lose more than 100 lbs. But I
will try to take this one step at a time, do it slowly, and stick to the

137

pattern I am creating for myself.

I will let you know on Tues. How the rest of the week goes. I am glad we are having more than one session as it helps us to follow up and gives us more reassurance to go forward. Build more strength as we go.

I remembered through the week   things you have said and of course it makes so much since. You are so right when you said , tell an overeater to eat 6 times a day. I agree 100% with everything that was taught to us on Tuesday, and I am so looking forward to the next session.

Thank you
Marj

Hi Jo-Anne,

I am so impressed! I've lost 4 lbs. in 4 days (since Tuesday, when I got weighed)

Thanks,
Maureen

I took the two-day Virtual Gastric Band training with Jo-Anne Eadie last weekend and loved every minute of it. Jo-Anne is empathetic, knowledgeable, likeable and warm. Her delivery is full of humor, clarity and focus. She is every bit a wonderful Hypnosis Trainer. I am excited about including this fabulous tool in my practice.

Yvonne

Hi Jo-Anne

Just wanted to say thank you for how great you've been with my parents and friends. They are all absolutely loving their experience with you (almost as much as me lol).

I was with Christa Monday night and we couldn't stop talking about how easy this is and how well it is working. Marjorie and Stephanie give me daily updates at work on how they feel and how amazing they think you are...which I totally agree with.

I love that I can share this experience with my parents as well. We are so close so the support we have for each other is really encouraging. I know those CDs will really help my mom...especially the affirmations. Who knows you might see my sister and her friends next, and then it'll be the whole Fletcher family. Ha-ha

The service you offer is fabulous and I will continue to advertise this to all I know with how well it's working. I'm still listening to the CDs...still only eating 3 meals a day. I have had a day or 2 where I wanted an afternoon snack, but I believe that was due to an insufficient breakfast. I certainly do have the sweet craving I once had. And trust me it was bad!

I'm glad our paths crossed when they did. Hope you have a good remainder of your week

Cheers

Amie

Hi Jo-Anne,

Thank you for the reminder. I have noted on my calendar that I have an appointment with you at 10:30am next Friday.

I wish to make you aware that I felt very at ease during my visit on Wednesday and now have only positive thoughts about my hypnotic journey with you to address my over-weight issues. You are a very gentle and kind person and I am pleased to be under your guidance. It is early days yet but you must have an initial report. I am listening to the tapes each day, reading your book, have posted the reminder posters in my kitchen and dining room, and am endeavouring to follow the daily three-meal regime.

I also wish to thank you for your gift of goodies and the recipes to enable me to bake my own. I enjoyed my first slice of the bread for breakfast Thursday morning and ate the muffin last evening. I am keeping a record of my queries and meals during this week in hope that we will have time to review them during our visit.

See you next Friday then,
Shirley

My Final Observations

I had my own Gastric band installed when my fellow hypnotist and I came home from the course and practiced on each other. I still feel it working and I can by-pass it, and I have on occasion, but I feel terrible.

One night we had hamburgers. We grow our own grass fed beef and the meat is wonderful. I add all my own ingredients and the hamburgers are yummy. I felt satisfied with one hamburger but ate a second one anyway. It just tasted so good.

My stomach felt stretched and I couldn't sit as I felt so uncomfortable. My stomach actually hurt. It made me examine what I was doing. Why did I go on eating when I felt satisfied? What had happened that day that perhaps triggered this?

There was nothing to "blame" it on except my **emotional integrity**. The days of self sabotage are over and I now realize a lot of reasons why I overeat, so who or what can I blame overeating on now? I can't – I need to have Emotional Integrity.

Going back to those old ways is allowing myself to again be a victim. I am not a victim. I was never a victim, I never want to again feel like or be a victim.

I know better now and I can't pretend that I don't.

That statement makes me feel better than any second helping, any sweet, any treat. Nothing tastes better than thin feels! Will I ever get off the train again – probably but I will get right back on.

Begin again – Finnegan

Bibliography

Look, Carol. "A Gratitude Experiment", www.attractingabundance.com, 2010

Hawkins, David. "Power vs. Force: The Hidden Determinations of Human Behaviou", 2002

Mercola, Dr. Joseph. "The Five Absolute Worst Foods You Can Eat", www.mercola.com, 2003

Nelson, Portia. "Autobiography in Five Short Chapters", 1993

Contact Jo-Anne Eadie

Jo-Anne Eadie
alkayjo@gmail.com

www.poweroffreedom.ca
www.aliencosmicexpo.com
www.canadianhypnosisconference.com

Linkedin:
https://ca.linkedin.com/in/jo-anne-eadie-61883b51

Youtube:
www.youtube.com/channel/UCHa3CucHW1BbkEp GpfvEL8w

www.ingramcontent.com/pod-product-compliance
Lightning Source LLC
Chambersburg PA
CBHW071324310526
45789CB00016B/609